Editors' Foreword

In most professions there is a traditional gulf between theory and its practice, and nursing is no exception. The gulf is perpetuated when theory is taught in a theoretical setting and practice is taught by the practitioner.

This inherent gulf has to be bridged by students of nursing, and publication of this series is an attempt to aid such bridge building.

It aims to help relate theory and practice in a meaningful way whilst underlining the importance of the person being cared for.

It aims to introduce students of nursing to some of the more common problems found in each new area of experience in which they will be asked to work.

It aims to de-mystify some of the technical language they will hear, putting it in context, giving it meaning and enabling understanding.

LEARNING TO CARE SERIES

General Editors

JEAN HEATH, BA, SRN, SCM, CERT ED
English National Board Learning Resources Unit,
Sheffield

SUSAN E NORMAN, SRN, DNCERT, RNT
Senior Tutor, The Nightingale School, West
Lambert Health Authority

Titles in this series include:

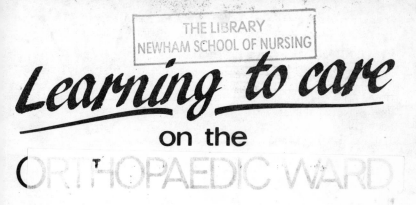

Learning to care

on the

ORTHOPAEDIC WARD

Danielle Julien
SRN, ONC, RNT

Nurse Tutor,
The Nightingale School,
St Thomas' Hospital

HODDER AND STOUGHTON
LONDON SYDNEY AUCKLAND TORONTO

LEARNING TO CARE SERIES

General Editors

JEAN HEATH, BA, SRN, SCM, CERT ED
English National Board Learning Resources Unit,
Sheffield

SUSAN E. NORMAN, SRN, DN CERT, RNT
Senior Tutor, The Nightingale School, West
Lambeth Health Authority

Titles in this series include:

Learning to Care for Elderly People
L. THOMAS
Learning to Care in the Community
P. TURTON and J. ORR
Learning to Care on the Medical Ward
A. MATTHEWS

British Library Cataloguing in Publication Data

Julien, Danielle
    Learning to care on the orthopaedic ward. –
    (Learning to care series)
    1. Orthopaedic nursing
    I. Title
    610.73'677   RD753

    ISBN 0 340 37061 0

First published 1986
Copyright © 1986 D. Julien

Typeset in 10/11pt Trump Mediaeval
by Rowland Phototypesetting Ltd,
Bury St Edmunds, Suffolk

Printed in Great Britain for
Hodder and Stoughton Educational,
a division of Hodder and Stoughton Ltd,
Mill Road, Dunton Green, Sevenoaks, Kent
TN13 2YD, by Richard Clay (The Chaucer Press) Ltd,
Bungay, Suffolk

Contents

Introduction

You are about to start work on an Orthopaedic ward. The people who are admitted to your ward will have neuro-musculo-skeletal disorders – bones broken or diseased, joints injured, muscles paralysed. These patients will be admitted to your ward either:

as an emergency due to trauma, e.g. a young man in a motor bike accident fractures his tibia and fibula, and may or may not have other life threatening injuries

or from the waiting list for conservative treatment or surgery, e.g.

a young woman suffering from a prolapsed intervertebral disc is admitted for bed rest before having a laminectomy.

The length of time a patient remains on the ward may vary from days to weeks or even months. The patient may have to have corrective surgery in years to come.

The equipment that you will see on the ward is often large and bulky. Do not be overawed by this. All the beds are of adjustable height and are equipped with wheels, a firm base and a lifting mechanism. These are ideal for moving a patient from the ward to a department for treatment. They can be fitted with a trapeze, better known as a monkey pole, which helps the patient maintain as much independence as possible whilst on bed rest.

Various appliances are used to immobilise or restrict movement either of the body or of a limb. Some appliances that you may see are:

Plaster of Paris casts
Splints

Functional bracing
Differing types of traction with or without pulley systems and beams
Walking aids such as walking frames, rollators, crutches, sticks and surgical shoes

If the patient is not allowed to bear weight or is unable to walk a wheelchair may be his only means of transport.

Bed making is unconventional in an orthopaedic ward because of the various appliances used. Bed clothes cover the patient but often do not look very tidy. The important point is to keep the patient comfortable and warm. Aids such as sheepskins, pillows and cradles, to mention a few, can be used to make life more tolerable for the patient.

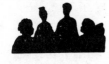

The nurse is an important and responsible part of the orthopaedic team. She works closely with doctors, physiotherapists, occupational therapists, radiologists, orthotists (splint and appliance makers), social workers, pharmacists, voluntary workers and relatives. She ensures that everyone knows what is happening (especially the patient!).

To do this she requires many skills. She must understand the neuro-musculo-skeletal system, how it works and what can go wrong. She needs interpersonal skills that develop trust and confidence in her patient and his relatives. She will use observational and technical skills, e.g. monitoring of vital signs, being acutely aware of the correct position of injured limbs and watchful for any deterioration such as numbness of the toes.

Whilst on the ward patients may undergo a variety of investigations of the neuro-musculo-skeletal system. Some investigations such as arthroscopy require the patient to be prepared for a general anaesthetic. Others such as a myelogram or radiculogram of the spine include the use of special X-rays.

Pre-operative check-list

The procedures for preparing a patient for theatre are the same on an orthopaedic ward as on other wards. The following is a general safety checklist.

Make sure the patient's medical notes and X-rays are ready to go with the patient to the theatre.

Ensure that the laboratory reports are present, particularly blood results of blood group, cross-matching, urea and electrolytes, and haemoglobin.

A consent form should be signed.

All jewellery, dentures, and contact lenses should be removed.

The patient should be wearing an operation gown.

Check that the patient has passed urine and note the amount.

Verify the patient's identity band against the notes and with the patient.

Ascertain that the correct premedication has been given at the right time.

Make notes of all proceedings in the nursing records.

| CARE |
| PLAN |

Following a general anaesthetic

On returning to the ward the nurse must watch for the following possible problems to which all patients who have had a general anaesthetic are susceptible.

Potential problem Acute respiratory obstruction may occur due to inhaled vomit or the tongue falling to the back of the throat.

Nursing care and rationale Ensure that the tongue is not occluding the airway. Observe the respiratory rate and watch for signs of obstruction, for example, shallow breathing, cyanosis, a rapid weak pulse and/or restlessness.

Potential problem Haemorrhage and/or haematoma formation may follow surgery and it is vital to maintain circulation and prevent shock.

Nursing care and rationale Examine the wound dressing for any obvious blood. Ensure that the vacuum drain is working properly, that the tube is not twisted or kinked and that the bottles are lower than the wound. Measure the fluid from the drain daily and report the amount on the fluid intake and output chart. If the vacuumed bottle is not working adequately, blood may ooze through the wound and soak the dressing or it may collect in the tissues resulting in a haematoma.

Take the pulse and blood pressure readings hourly until they are stable. Fluctuations in these will alert you to changes in the patient's cardiac function and output and should be reported immediately to the person in charge of the ward.

Actual problem Pain due to surgery must be relieved or prevented to improve the patient's recovery rate.

Nursing care and rationale Analgesia will be given as prescribed by the doctor usually 4- or 6-hourly whenever necessary. Pain may be due to swelling, for example a tight feeling around the joint arising from poor positioning of the limb. Research findings suggest that if a patient's pain is well controlled then recovery is quicker.

Jennifer Bloore (1979) suggests that preparing a patient pre-operatively and explaining that analgesia is available following surgery will enable that patient to cope with the pain. However the nurse must assess and plan with the patient the amount of analgesia to be given.

From the moment the patient is admitted the orthopaedic nurse commences the rehabilitative process. Always allow patients to do as much for themselves as they can. They must be independent in order to cope with the activities of living and eventually resume a normal life. It does not matter if the patient is slow; always praise what has been achieved.

Other members of the team play a very important role in the patient's rehabilitation. The physiotherapist, whilst treating the patient on the ward, might also wish the patient to visit the department for further treatment. The latter helps in the patient's rehabilitation by widening his horizons.

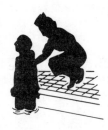

One form of treatment which can be used to increase mobility is hydrotherapy, during which patients are able to exercise in water. The warmth and buoyancy of the water causes relaxation, reduces pain and allows the patient to achieve a greater range of movement than on dry land. The hospital you are working in, however, may not have a hydrotherapy pool.

To maintain the patients' well being the nurse must constantly assess and evaluate their needs. Your patient is often not 'ill' but constrained by some injury and the various appliances mentioned above. People with an active mind may well become bored and frustrated with these constraints. They may be fretful or worried about commitments in the outside world which are being neglected. The nurse must at all times be alert and aware that enforced bed rest can make the patient socially isolated. Restlessness, confusion, hostility, disorientation and the inability to concentrate are signs of sensory deprivation. The nurse must assess each situation and plan an individual programme of care to ensure that the patient is stimulated. Throughout their stay in hospital patients can take an active role in planning their care. The nurse can help the patient come to terms with and overcome both temporary and long-term restrictions on his freedom.

The orthopaedic patient is rewarding to nurse. Once over the initial trauma the patient's condition improves with time allowing the nurse to develop and establish a good working relationship, sharing both tragedy and triumph.

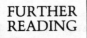

FURTHER READING

BLOORE, J. 1979. Nursing Surgical Patients in Acute Pain. *Nursing*, 1st series, April, **1**, 37–43.
HAYWARD, J. 1975. *Information – a Prescription against Pain*. London: RCN.

2 Mrs Beech, a housewife with a back problem

Mrs Beech is a 36 year old housewife. Her husband is a sales representative and they live in a semi-detached house with two small children: Christopher aged 5 years and Ian, aged 3 years. It was at Ian's birthday party that Mrs Beech hurt her back. She was bending over to pick him up when she felt a sharp pain in the small of her back. The pain radiated down her right leg. The pain was so acute that Mrs Beech was unable to move and was forced to stand in a tilted position for some time. Her husband was so worried that he called their general practitioner who had her admitted to the local hospital. Following the doctor's examination Mrs Beech was diagnosed as suffering from a prolapsed intervertebral disc.

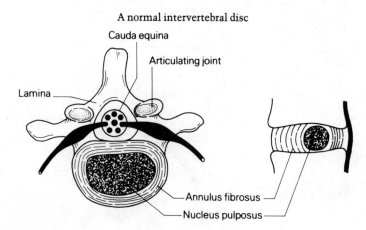

A normal intervertebral disc

Cauda equina

Articulating joint

Lamina

Annulus fibrosus

Nucleus pulposus

General causes of back pain:
Trauma – accidents, strains and very poor lifting technique
Disorder of the spinal cord, e.g. tumour
Osteoarthrosis of the articulating joint.
Congenital abnormality of the vertebrae
Referred pain from diseases in the abdominal cavity e.g. kidney infections

In 1981 the Materials Handling Research Unit at the University of Surrey reported that their survey showed that 40 000 nurses hurt their back each year.

The Back Pain Association and the Materials Handling Research Unit estimate that 20 million working days are lost each year because of back pain.

What is a prolapsed intervertebral disc?

The spine (vertebral column) consists of bones (vertebrae) which extend from the neck (cervical) region through the back (thoracic) region to the lower back (lumbar and saccral) region. Each vertebrae is held in place by many ligaments. This pillar of bones forms a continuous column which houses the spinal cord in its centre. The spinal cord extends from the medulla oblongata in the brain to the level of lumbar 1–2. Here it forms a collection of nerves called the cauda equina. In between the vertebrae there are rings of fibrocartilage called intervertebral discs. Each disc consists of an outer fibrous ring, the annulus fibrosus, and a central gelatinous mass

Nerve compressed on one side causing pain and sciatica

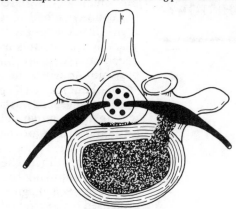

Central disc protrusion causing back ache

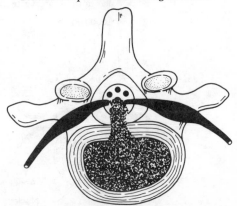

called the nucleus pulposus. Both have no nerve supply. When trauma occurs to the back, e.g. lifting a heavy weight with the back flexed, the strain causes the annulus fibrosus to tear allowing the nucleus pulposus to move forward into the vertebral canal. This causes pressure on the spinal cord or its collection of nerves, leading to acute back pain.

ADMISSION TO THE WARD

On arrival on the ward Mrs Beech is apprehensive and in pain, and her husband is anxious and worried. After the nurse introduces herself as Christine and welcomes Mrs Beech to the ward, she explains that Mrs Beech is to be nursed flat in bed on pelvic traction as prescribed by her doctor. This traction is used to increase the space between the vertebrae and therefore relieve the pressure on the nerve, reducing pain. Mrs Beech will remain on pelvic traction for two weeks. It was explained to her by her consultant that every 6 hours she would receive analgesia for the pain, and sedation to cause relaxation of the muscle spasm.

What is pelvic traction?
Pelvic traction consists of a well fitting pelvic belt made of canvas to which are attached straps leading to cord and weights.

Pelvic traction for low back pain

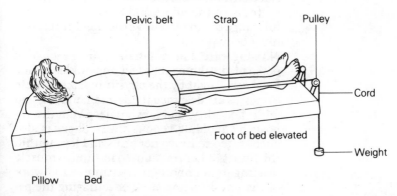

Body weight = counter traction

Whilst admitting Mrs Beech Christine discovered that she was very anxious about her children and her husband. She was reassured when reminded that her retired mother-in-law had agreed to come and stay with the children. Christine also told her of the visiting hours and arranged that the children could visit her. It is important that the patient is psychologically as well as physically at rest, to promote the relaxation that will aid her recovery.

CARE PLAN for Mrs Beech whilst on bed rest

Actual problem Pain from the nerve compression has to be modified and relieved.
Nursing care and rationale Analgesics and a sedative were given 6-hourly to control her pain and relax muscle spasm. Mrs Beech was encouraged to describe to Christine exactly what pain she felt as she may have moved in the bed and caused the pelvic sling to be badly aligned, thus increasing the pain.
Evaluation Mrs Beech said that her pain was well controlled and always pointed out to the nurses if her straps were twisted.

Potential problem Immobility due to pelvic traction and enforced bed rest may lead to stiffness of the joints and muscle wasting. A full range of movement within her limitations must be maintained.
Nursing care and rationale Mrs Beech was persuaded to move her feet and ankles as she had been taught by the physiotherapist. These exercises are designed to maintain muscle and joint flexibility, and prevent deep vein thrombosis by avoiding venous stasis. She was also encouraged to move her arms and legs within the limits of her traction, to minimise muscle wasting. It is important to reinforce the work of the physiotherapist by encouraging the patient to exercise.

Evaluation Mrs Beech enjoyed her exercises which she did for five minutes every hour whilst she was awake. Thus she maintained mobility and avoided stiffness.

Ankle Exercises

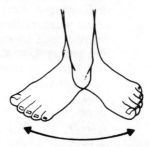

1 Turn both feet inwards and outwards as far as possible

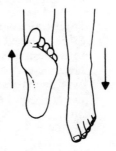

2 Point your feet down and then point your toes up

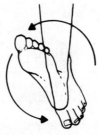

3 Circle your feet in a clockwise direction and then in an anti-clockwise direction.

Potential problem Boredom because of the enforced bed rest has to be avoided and she should be encouraged to retain interest in herself, her family and observe the goings on in the ward.

Nursing care and rationale Mrs Beech's mother-in-law drew up a visiting plan so that there were visitors at regular intervals. This stimulated Mrs Beech's interest in herself and her family. Christine distracted her by providing reading material from the hospital library together with a reading frame and mirror. She also wheeled Mrs Beech into the day room on her bed to allow her to watch television.

Evaluation Mrs Beech appeared withdrawn sometimes. Christine found that spending a few moments talking with her from time to time helped restore Mrs Beech to her usual happy and cheerful self.

Potential problem Anorexia may arise as it is difficult to eat and drink while lying down. She must be encouraged to take nourishment.

Nursing care and rationale Christine offered Mrs Beech the menu card and helped her to choose small appetising meals as she felt full after just a few mouthfuls. It was also suggested to her mother-in-law that Mrs Beech's favourite foods could be brought in to entice her to eat a balanced diet. Flexible straws were provided to help her to drink without spilling.

Evaluation Christine ascertained that Mrs Beech was having a well balanced diet by watching what she ate at meal times. Mrs Beech particularly liked to share her food with her children as this gave the meal a family atmosphere. However, she often complained of indigestion and a very full feeling after eating only a little food.

Potential problem Urinary elimination is difficult when lying flat, and urinary stasis, leading to urinary tract infection and the possible formation of renal calculi, must be prevented.

Nursing care and rationale Mrs Beech was unable to use a female urinal but coped with the slipper bed pan. She was encouraged to drink 3 litres daily through flexistraws as a large fluid intake helps to prevent urinary stasis. An accurate fluid intake and output chart must be kept and the colour of her urine noted. Dark coloured urine is concentrated, usually as a result of the patient not drinking enough. Fishy smelling urine indicates a urinary infection.

Evaluation After Mrs Beech became accustomed to the slipper bed pan, no difficulties were encountered. She enjoyed a variety of drinks both hot and cold.

Potential problem Constipation and flatulence due to immobility can be avoided by promoting bowel action.

Nursing care and rationale Mrs Beech was encouraged to eat a high fibre diet including tomatoes, lettuce, bran and prune juice.

Evaluation Good bowel habits were maintained throughout her stay. Mrs Beech was convinced that this was due to the prune juice that she had each morning at breakfast time.

Actual problem She is unable to wash herself properly whilst on traction, and thus sores must be prevented and freshness, cleanliness and patient dignity promoted.

Nursing care and rationale Mrs Beech needed a great deal of time to wash her face, arms and chest as she tired easily. Her pelvic belt and the padding under the length of the belt was undone to wash and examine the skin. The padding prevents the belt from digging into the skin and causing pressure sores. Talc was applied sparingly under the belt as patients wearing a canvas pelvic corset often become hot and sweaty, but too much talc can cake and abrade the skin. She cleaned her own teeth but found this very difficult. The situation improved when using a flexistraw to rinse her mouth and spit into a receiver. Her hair was washed weekly.

Evaluation Her skin remained in good condition. Her pressure points were observed daily, but no skin abrasions or sores developed. She did not complain of pain in her leg or lower back while she remained on pelvic traction. She was allowed to move in bed within the limits of her traction.

The pressure points

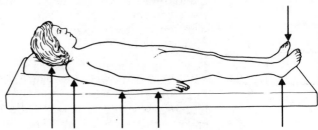

Patient lying supine

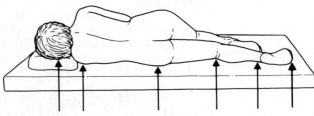

Patient lying on side

<table>
<tr><td>NURSING
CARE</td></tr>
</table>

Initial Stages

After two weeks on bed rest, Mrs Beech was taken off pelvic traction on her doctor's instructions. Before she was allowed to stand, a corset (lumbar support) was made for her. This had to be worn at all times when out of bed, to prevent lumbar flexion. The physiotherapist taught Mrs Beech to stand correctly and each day she was able to stand for longer periods.

As the days went by Mrs Beech found walking difficult as she seemed unable to lift her right foot off the ground. She was terribly upset; she became weepy and believed she would never be well again. Christine arranged for her doctor to come and see her as soon as possible and he ordered a radiculogram. A straight X-ray of the spine would not show the tearing of the disc as there is no narrowing of the space between the intervertebral discs. This narrowing will only occur when the disc has disintegrated.

NURSING CARE

Diagnosis

Christine explained to Mrs Beech that she was to have an X-ray of her back (spine). She could eat a light meal and drink normally before this test. A dye would be injected into her lower back in the X-ray Department. The X-ray table then tilts to the required position and pictures of the spine taken. This procedure would last for 2 hours. Christine also emphasised that on her return to the ward Mrs Beech would have to stay in a sitting position for 6 hours but that she would be able to eat and drink during that time.

What is a radiculogram?
This is an invasive procedure used where other methods have failed to show the cause of the back pain. A dye is injected, by means of a lumbar puncture, into the sub-arachnoid space. An X-ray is then taken of the spine and it will show any obstruction in the spinal cord, e.g. PID or tumour. The term radiculogram is used when the lower nerve roots of the spinal cord are being examined. A myelogram refers to examination of the spinal cord as high as the cervical region. *If the dye is water soluble the patient must sit up for 6 hours. The dye must not be allowed to flow upwards as it may cause cerebral meningitis. The nurse should observe for signs of meningeal irritation: photophobia, diplopia,*

restlessness, vomiting, headache and elevated temperature. The X-ray department will give instructions on the type of dye used and the length of time the patient must remain upright.

What is a laminectomy?
Laminectomy means removal of the lamina. At operation the surgeon excises the ligament and removes part of the lamina. The protruding part of the disc is also removed.

After her radiculogram it was found that Mrs Beech had a prolapsed intervertebral disc at the level of lumbar spine vertebrae 4 and 5. She discussed this with her doctor and her husband. It was decided jointly that Mrs Beech would undergo a laminectomy and removal of disc.

Before the operation Christine ensured that both Mr and Mrs Beech understood what would happen. She explained that she would have a surgical dressing on her lower back, with a wound drain attached to a vacuum bottle. This drains away excess blood, so preventing a haematoma at her operation site. It was quite a normal procedure and the drain

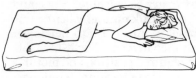

a

Lying on side, 1 pillow under head, 1 pillow under leg.

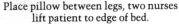

b

Place pillow between legs, two nurses lift patient to edge of bed.

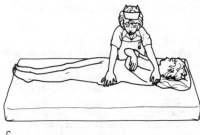

c

Nurse places one hand on shoulder, and one hand on buttock. Patient turns head in direction of move, folds arms across chest and crosses ankles. Move in one.

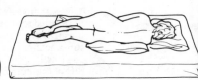

d

Replace pillows. Log roll completed.

would be removed after two days. Her sutures would be taken out after ten days. Analgesia will be given regularly for her pain.

As after the operation Mrs Beech would not be able to sit up and would have to lie on her side, the nurse taught her now how to 'log roll' from side to side to avoid skin breakdown over pressure points.

Mrs Beech was thankful that she knew what would happen but was anxious about her anaesthetic – would she wake up after the operation? Christine reassured her by contacting the anaesthetist who came to talk to both Mrs Beech and her husband.

An alternative method of 'log rolling' a patient:
A draw sheet can be used to turn the patient. Loosen the drawsheet on both sides. Ask the patient to cross arms across the chest, keep legs straight and face the opposite side. Two nurses pull the drawsheet on the opposite side to the one on which the patient will end up facing. This will roll the patient.

This type of drawsheet 'log rolling' is most effective if the patient has been taught it prior to operation; however, dragging of the patient may occur and thus two nurses are required for the move.

Mrs Beech was prepared for theatre as for any other surgical procedure.

CARE PLAN

for Mrs Beech following her laminectomy

Potential problem Enforced bed rest following surgery must not lead to dependence on nursing ministrations, and independence must be encouraged.
Nursing care and rationale Mrs Beech remained on flat bed rest for two weeks. Correct alignment of the spine is necessary as any bending would cause strain and prevent healing of the tissues. After this time she was allowed to either stand (providing she was wearing her corset) or to lie down, but not to sit

up. She was turned from side to side by log rolling every two hours or earlier if she felt the need to move.

Evaluation Two weeks later she was seen by the physiotherapist and commenced mobilisation. After 5 days of this she was able to do so without assistance.

Potential problem The complications of bed rest (which are: chest infection, deep vein thrombosis, and urinary retention) must be prevented.

Nursing care and rationale Repeatedly remind her of her deep breathing exercises as these increase lung expansion. Otherwise, secretions may collect in the alveolar sacs and possibly become infected.

Encourage ankle and foot exercises as stasis of blood in the veins can lead to deep vein thrombosis. The formation of a clot may be discovered by observing any swelling, pain, tenderness and raised skin temperature in the affected calf. Take 4-hourly observations of temperature, pulse and respiration. An elevation of temperature takes place normally after 48 hours because of the inflammatory response to the incision. Verify that Mrs Beech has sensation in her lower legs. Observe for any numbness or tingling and if the situation worsens inform the doctor.

Report any failure to void urine as the operation can disrupt the nerve supplying the bladder and thereby urinary retention can occur. A fluid intake and output chart kept for 48 hours will either confirm or dispel suspicions of retention.

Evaluation Mrs Beech produced no cough or sputum. No signs of deep vein thrombosis were reported. Her urinary output totalled 1500 to 3500 ml per 24 hours.

Planning discharge

Mrs Beech made a splendid recovery. She had no pain either in her leg or back. She was seen by Jane the occupational therapist who gave her various aids so that she could look after herself without bending too far: a stocking aid, a shoe horn, a 'helping hand', and a raised toilet seat.

Before going home Christine gave Mrs Beech a list of do's and don'ts:

Do	continue with the back exercises and abdominal exercises to strengthen the lumbar spine
Do	bend knees and hips when lifting
Do	stand or sit with your back straight – good posture
Do	lie on your side with knees bent
Do	rest if you feel tired
Do	remain at your ideal weight – obesity produces bad posture
Do	walk each day – exercise is good for you
DO NOT	bend at the waist

After Mrs Beech had read her list with her husband she had a few questions:

Could she drive a car?

She was not allowed to drive the car for the first month to six weeks. This is because of the possible strain on the back when getting out of the car and sitting for long periods in traffic queues.

What about housework?

She was told not to recommence housework for one month and then to use the techniques which she had been taught by the occupational therapist and physiotherapist.

She felt that she would wear her corset until she became more confident with her exercises. She was also still anxious whether the pain would return. The nurse assured her that providing that she followed the list of do's and don'ts there was no reason why she should not make a complete recovery.

Mrs Beech was given a follow-up appointment in 6 weeks' time and discharged home. Her mother-in-law stayed for a further month with the family until it was felt that they could all cope.

TEST YOURSELF

1 What are the main causes of prolapsed intervertebral disc?

2 What is the purpose of pelvic traction?

3 Why was a laminectomy performed?

4 Why was the nurse concerned about Mrs Beech's urinary output?

5 What role does the physiotherapist play in Mrs Beech's care?

6 What part did the various members of the orthopaedic team play in Mrs Beech's care?

7 What role did the occupational therapist play in Mrs Beech's discharge?

8 What role did Mrs Beech's family play in aiding recovery?

FURTHER READING

CRAWFORD ADAMS, J. 1981. *Outline of Orthopaedics*, 9th ed. Edinburgh: Churchill Livingstone.
FARRELL, J. 1982. *Illustrated Guide to Orthopedic Nursing*, 2nd ed. Philadelphia: Lippincott.
MAY, J. 1979. Low Back Pain – A Care Study. *Nursing* 1 (3), 132–4. June.
POWELL, M. 1982. *Orthopaedic Nursing and Rehabilitation*, 8th ed. Edinburgh: Churchill Livingstone.
ROAF, R. AND HODKINSON, L. 1980. *Textbook of Orthopaedic Nursing*, 3rd ed. Oxford: Blackwell Scientific Publications.
TROUP, D. *et al.* (Eds). 1981. *The Handling of Patients – A Guide for Nurse Managers*. London: Royal College of Nursing, Back Pain Association.

3 Mrs Neilson, a widow with osteoarthrosis of her hip

Mrs Neilson is 65 years of age, and has been a widow for five years. She lives in a bungalow by the sea, and her son lives nearby while her married daughter lives 100 miles away.

She is an energetic lady with many friends and is often seen walking her dog Rebel, a Labrador. Since her retirement she liked to take Rebel for a walk along the sea front. Lately though, she has found that walking produces pain in her left hip. This pain becomes so severe that she has to stop walking and sit down and rest. After a short time the pain lessens and she can walk again after a momentary stiffness. She attributed this pain to 'getting old' and that it must be 'rheumatism'.

However as time went by and the pain in her left hip worsened, Mrs Neilson went to see her General Practitioner. Examination revealed stiffness in moving her hip, with a creaking sound. The doctor sent Mrs Neilson to the local hospital for an X-ray.

On her return visit to discuss the results, the doctor told her that she had osteoarthrosis of her left hip.

What is osteoarthrosis?

This condition is also known as degenerative arthritis and as osteoarthritis. Both are misnomers as no inflammation actually takes place. Osteoarthrosis is a degenerative disorder which arises in a synovial joint. The primary cause is unknown but it occurs with advancing years. However age, sex, heredity, secondary obesity and mechanical stress to the joint may be predisposing factors.

21

What changes occur at a synovial joint?

The articular cartilage becomes roughened and cracks. This cartilage wears away leaving bare bone. The cracking of the bone causes stress and therefore new bone is produced where articular cartilage should be, forming bony out-growths (osteophytes). The wearing away of bone is progressive and eventually the whole articulating surface is destroyed. Joint space is lost and movement at that joint is extremely painful.

A normal synovial joint

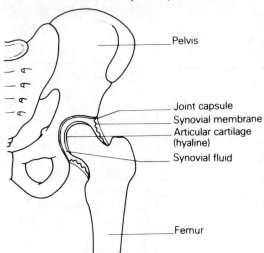

Pelvis

Joint capsule
Synovial membrane
Articular cartilage
(hyaline)
Synovial fluid

Femur

Changes occurring in osteoarthrosis

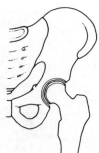

Thinning articular cartilage

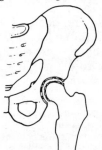

Cracking of articular cartilage

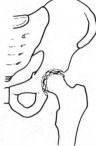

New bone growth (osteophytes) causing pain and loss of movement

Joints affected in
osteoarthrosis are
mainly weight-
bearing: hip, knee,
ankle and spine.

Joints affected in
osteoarthrosis are
mainly weight-
bearing: hip, knee,
ankle and spine.

In non-weight
bearing joints, e.g.
the shoulder,
though the disease
process may be
seen on X-ray, the
patient does not
complain of any
symptoms.

What are the symptoms of osteoarthrosis?

1 Pain on movement and especially in cold weather.
2 Stiffness of the joint when rested and when
   movement is recommenced.
3 Creaking and grinding of the joint (crepitus).
4 The patient tires very quickly with the exertion of
   walking.
5 Bony enlargement of the fingers (Heberden's nodes).

The doctor explained to Mrs Neilson that he
could give her some tablets to relieve the pain
but that she could help herself by taking frequent rest periods. It is bearing weight on an
osteoarthritic joint that causes pain and it is
best relieved by rest. He also arranged for her to
see the domiciliary occupational therapist for
home assessment and the physiotherapist for
an exercise programme. The doctor reassured
Mrs Neilson that although the disease can be
crippling for some people, others manage very
well with this regime.

The doctor explained that he would pre-
scribe Paracetamol tablets, two to be taken
every four or six hours when necessary. He
suggested that Mrs Neilson take two tablets
with her morning cup of tea, to start the day,
and two tablets at night, so as to have a good
night's sleep.

NURSING CARE

Initial stages

Mrs Neilson was also seen by Jane, the occupational therapist, who came to see her at
home. As Mrs Neilson lived in a bungalow,
Jane found things well laid out. However they
discussed the following points which ought to
minimise the pain in her hip by taking some of
the strain off the joint and enable her to maintain her independence.

In the kitchen:
To sit while preparing her meals and when

doing the ironing. This will relieve stress from prolonged standing on her hip.

To use two hands when lifting any kitchen equipment and to have every day equipment at hand and within easy reach.

To use a long-handled dustpan and brush.

In the bathroom:
   a non-slip mat in the bath
   bathboard and seat
   raised toilet seat

After this discussion on the provision of aids Jane felt that Mrs Neilson was much happier with how she was going to cope at home. Mrs Neilson also knew that she could contact Jane whenever she felt she needed more help.

Mrs Neilson then visited the Physiotherapy Department. There she met Mary who talked about the following points and taught her these exercises:

1 Good posture is extremely important as it will minimise pain and prevent deformity. When walking or climbing stairs as well as standing, Mrs Neilson should put her shoulders back and think tall so as to keep her body in alignment. Also she ought to sit straight.

2 Use a warm hot water bottle to relieve pain in the hip. Mrs Neilson was told never to put the hot water bottle directly on her skin as she could burn herself but to put a cover over the bottle or wrap it in a towel.

3 These following exercises are important as they stabilise the pelvis when weight is taken on the leg. Mrs Neilson was taught to lie flat on her back (supine) and on her tummy (prone) with her legs slightly apart (abducted). This she did for one hour each day to correct any deformity occurring at the hip which could stop her from walking.

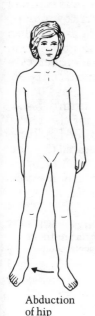

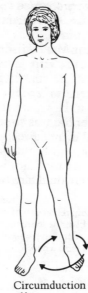

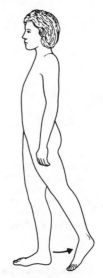

Abduction of hip	Circumduction of hip	Extension of hip

Mrs Neilson managed very well at home taking her Paracetamol tablets, having two in the morning and two in the evening. She also took two tablets before walking Rebel. She found that this routine controlled her pain well. She still walked along the sea front but took frequent rests along the promenade, making use of the benches. Here with these frequent stops she made friends with the other people walking their dogs.

She found invaluable the help that Jane had given her as she now did not get tired during the day. However as time went by she was less able to straighten her left hip. Her tablets had been changed several times from Paracetamol to Aspirin then to distalgesics and finally to Paramol. However even these were now no longer effective and she was in constant pain. Mrs Neilson was unable to meet her friends because walking for any distance was painful. Therefore she also could not do her own shopping. She felt as though she might as well give up.

Seeing Mrs Neilson becoming more depressed on each visit, her doctor sent her to see an orthopaedic consultant. Several X-rays of her hip were taken and her osteoarthrosis was found to be worse. The consultant also noted that her hip was so stiff that it could hardly be moved in any direction. He suggested that she have a total hip replacement. With this operation her mobility would be greatly restored and she would have little or no pain.

A prosthesis is an artificial substitute used to replace a missing body part e.g. head of femur removed, artificial product made to take its place.

What is a total hip replacement?

A total hip replacement involves removing the ball (head and neck) of the femur and inserting a stem prosthesis into the femur in its place. The socket (acetabulum) is replaced with a cup.

Diseased joint showing head of femur and acetabulum merging

Total hip replacement

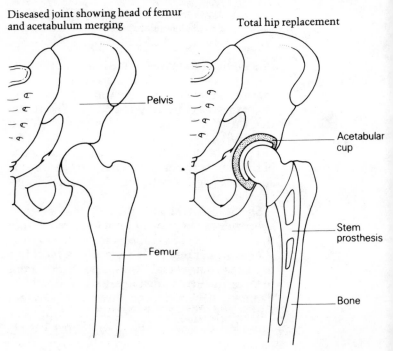

Pelvis

Acetabular cup

Stem prosthesis

Femur

Bone

The orthopaedic consultant told Mrs Neilson that she would be admitted within the next few months. He reassured her that all should go well and she would be in hospital between two and three weeks, and she returned home to ponder this new change in her treatment.

ADMISSION TO THE WARD

On arrival at the hospital 48 hours before her operation, Mrs Neilson was welcomed by Jenny Bell, the ward sister, who showed her to her bed and introduced her to student nurse, Christine Wolf.

Christine welcomed Mrs Neilson warmly and introduced her to the other patients in her bay. As it was noon Christine offered her some lunch before admitting her.

Then she recorded Mrs Neilson's temperature, pulse, respirations, blood pressure, weight and height. These 'normal' observations provide a baseline for later assessment.

While Christine was taking these observations she spoke to Mrs Neilson about what was going to happen during her stay in hospital. This put Mrs Neilson at ease and made her less anxious, and it gave her the opportunity to ask questions. Mrs Neilson remarked that though she missed Rebel and knew that he would pine for her, she was happy that her son and daughter-in-law were able to look after him.

Christine explained that her operation would be in two days time but before that various tests had to be done pre-operatively.

The tests were:
1 Blood tests. Blood would be taken for haemoglobin estimation to see if she was anaemic. Her blood would also be grouped and cross matched as it was possible that she would need a blood transfusion.
2 X-rays would be taken of her chest and her hip. The former would be used by the anaesthetist to ensure that all was well with her lungs and the latter by the surgeon to estimate the damage to the hip and to measure for the prothesis that he was going to use.

3   The Houseman and the anaesthetist would come to see her to check that all was well. They would ask if she had false teeth and if she was allergic to anything at all, especially elastoplast and penicillin. The houseman would take an ECG (electrocardiogram), a routine test for anyone over the age of 60 having an operation. Also he would ask her about her past medical history.
4   The physiotherapist would visit Mrs Neilson to teach her some deep breathing exercises. These exercises prevent stasis of the blood and reduce the risk of clot formation and pulmonary embolism postoperatively.

Christine then explained to Mrs Neilson that her consultant liked all his patients to be nursed with their leg in a foam trough. This prevents the leg from being adducted inadvertently, e.g. crossing her legs during sleep, and thus dislocating the hip. Another method used to achieve this is the use of abduction pillows. Christine said that the leg would be kept in this trough for four days and five nights. Mrs Neilson would also wear anti-embolitic stockings to aid venous return.

Foam trough

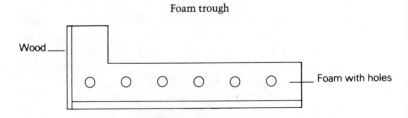

Wood

Foam with holes

Mrs Neilson thanked Christine for her explanation. She asked if her son and daughter could visit her on the day of her operation. Christine explained to Mrs Neilson that she would be very sleepy on that day because of the anaesthetic drugs. It would be best for them to telephone the ward first, because each person reacts differently to anaesthesia. Christine was aware while she was speaking that Mrs Neilson was anxious and apprehensive about her operation. She made a mental note to report this to the ward sister and the other nurses at the time of the report that afternoon and to note it in Mrs Neilson's care plan. Christine continued talking as she was filling in the history. Mrs Neilson mentioned that she really missed her dog and she knew she was silly to feel like this as he would be well looked after by her son. Christine encouraged her to talk about Rebel and looked at some photographs that Mrs Neilson had brought into hospital with her.

From midnight the evening before her operation Mrs Neilson had nothing to eat or drink. This reduces the risk of her inhaling vomit postoperatively. In the morning, using the antiseptic lotion which Christine had given her, Mrs Neilson had her bath whilst the other patients were eating their breakfasts. Meanwhile Christine made up her bed with clean linen. She also put in a bed cradle as this would be needed after the operation to keep the bed clothes off the operated leg. She ascertained that a monkey pole was attached.

The bed was ready for Mrs Neilson to be taken in it to the operating theatre. All the equipment would be in place ready for when she came out of the theatre. The houseman came around and marked her left leg with an arrow to ensure that the correct leg was operated on.

Mrs Neilson wore a hospital theatre gown. Christine checked she was not wearing any jewellery or make-up or dentures and that she had passed urine. She also made sure that the identity bracelet had the correct information, that Mrs Neilson had signed her consent form. Her premedication was given one hour before the operation, together with her first dose of antibiotics. She was told that the premedication would make her sleepy and her mouth dry. Antibiotics were given prophylactically to prevent joint infection (septic arthritis).

Christine ensured that Mrs Neilson's notes and X-rays went to the theatre with her.

Rehabilitation

On her return to the ward, the recovery nurse told Christine that Mrs Neilson had had a left total hip replacement as planned, and that her observations were stable. Mrs Neilson's operated leg was in a foam trough. She had two vacuum drains from her hip wound to prevent haematoma formation and reduce the risk of wound infection. An intravenous infusion of normal saline would run for a day or two to replace fluids lost during the operation. Though very sleepy, she recognised Christine and gave her a smile. Christine told her that she was back on the ward, and that her observations would be taken frequently and that all was normal.

Mrs Neilson could feel Christine touching her leg and asked what she was doing. Christine explained, 'Checking the wound dressing and the pulse in your foot' (pedal pulse). She looked at the wound dressing for any bleeding or oozing and felt the pedal pulse to determine if there was impaired circulation as a result of the surgical procedure. Christine compared the pedal pulse in the right leg with that in the opposite leg.

for Mrs Neilson postoperatively

Potential problem Dislocation of the hip due to improper positioning or movement of the left leg.

Nursing care and rationale Ensure that her left leg remains slightly abducted in the foam trough and do not allow her to sit up to more than 45 degrees of hip flexation. Violent flex-ation of the hip can cause its dislocation. Do not turn her on her side unless ordered by the consultant. Check any sudden severe pain that she may have, as it may indicate that the hip is dislocated. Once healing of the tissues has taken place, it is unlikely that the hip will become dislocated.

Evaluation Mrs Neilson was allowed to sit up to 45 degrees of hip flexion. She used the leg trough for 4 days and nights and was dis-appointed when it was removed. She told Christine, 'I felt safe with the trough as I knew that with it I was unable to cross my legs. Now I feel vulnerable.' Christine reminded her that she was progressing well.

A check X-ray was scheduled for the second day. Mrs Neilson was transported to the X-ray Department on her bed. The X-ray showed that all was well, and Mrs Neilson was not complaining of any pain postoperatively. She told Christine, 'The pain in my hip was so bad before that the pain of this operation is nothing by comparison! It just feels wonderful that I can move this leg.'

Potential problem Inactivity may lead to venous stasis and thence to deep vein throm-bosis. A deep vein thrombosis can be fatal if the patient has a pulmonary embolus.

Nursing care and rationale Mrs Neilson will wear anti-embolitic stockings on both legs immediately postoperatively. Ankle and leg movements suggested by the physiotherapist are to be encouraged to prevent venous stasis (see p. 11). Remember to remove anti-embolitic stockings daily to check the state of the skin.

Evaluation Mrs Neilson liked her anti-embolitic stockings. She said that it was just like wearing strong support stockings or tights. (Some patients may also have anticoagulant drugs prescribed by the doctor. These drugs would usually be administered prophylactically.)

Potential problem Inactivity may cause her to not breathe very deeply which could lead to chest infection and then to pneumonia.

Nursing care and rationale Encourage Mrs Neilson to take deep breaths and to continue with her deep breathing exercises. She should be seen by the physiotherapist daily.

Evaluation Mrs Neilson did her deep breathing exercises several times during the day. She did not have a cough.

Potential problem Her enforced bed rest may lead to the development of pressure sores.

Nursing care and rationale Change Mrs Neilson's position four-hourly, ensuring that she does not bend her hip more than 45 degrees. Check the skin over pressure points (see Chapter 2). Place a sheepskin under the heel of the unaffected leg and/or under her bottom, whichever suits the patient.

Moving a patient hourly, two-hourly or four-hourly is essential as the pressure of bone, e.g. hip bones, through to the skin causes the tissues in between to become ischaemic and tearing of the tissues can occur.

Evaluation Mrs Neilson complained of a very sore bottom to Christine, and it looked red and grazed. Mrs Neilson was shown how to use the 'monkey pole' to relieve the pressure on her bottom. It was her salvation she said.

Christine had used Dermalex solution on Mrs Neilson's bottom but when it became very red, Christine discontinued the use of the solution. Excessive use of Dermalex can in itself cause redness.

Mrs Neilson also found that the bottom exercises which the physiotherapist had taught her were helpful, e.g. squeeze buttocks together as hard as she can and then release.

Mrs Neilson had an intravenous infusion when she returned to the ward. This infusion had been used in the theatre to give her some blood as she had lost a certain amount during the operation. However, it was discontinued as soon as she was able to drink normally. Mrs Neilson had no major complications. She was able to maintain her own hygiene except for the affected leg.

From the time that Mrs Neilson first got out of bed until her discharge, the physiotherapist gave her a planned programme of mobility exercises.

On the second day postoperatively Mrs Neilson stood up with the assistance of the physiotherapist. Before this Christine had given Mrs Neilson some analgesia. Mrs Neilson said that she felt a little giddy and held on to the zimmer frame that was in front of her. The giddiness quickly passed and she was returned to bed, delighted with her achievement of the day. So much so in fact that she rang her son and daughter to tell them the news.

During the following days Mrs Neilson performed exercises to strengthen the hip and knee muscles of both legs. These included flexing the knee and the hip but keeping the operated leg abducted. Extreme hip flexion was avoided on the left leg.

Mrs Neilson soon became adept at getting out of bed. Her left leg was held in an abducted position while she moved her left hip to the side of the bed. She then put her operated leg on the floor. Lowering her right leg to the floor, Mrs Neilson then straightened up using the zimmer frame.

She spent one hour each afternoon lying prone to prevent hip flexion deformity. While in bed she liked having the back rest during the day and preferred just two pillows at night. She found that her left leg would swell by the end of the day, so Christine ensured that her anti-embolitic stocking fitted properly, and that she elevated her left leg on a stool when sitting in a chair.

After that there was no holding Mrs Neilson. She improved in leaps and bounds. She followed the physiotherapist's instructions. She walked with her walking frame, progressed to two sticks and then to one stick. The sutures were removed on the tenth day. She managed the stairs on day 14 and she was then discharged home.

NURSING CARE

Planning discharge

Before going home she was given an instruction sheet by the occupational therapist who had seen her in the department for an assessment of how she would cope at home. She was told to continue to use her raised toilet seat. Arrangements were made for a grab rail to be fitted in her bathroom.

Advice to Mrs Neilson

For the first three months to reduce the risk of dislocation of the hip:

Do not cross your legs.

Do not sit on low chairs. Choose high firm upright chairs. Put your affected leg slightly forward when you wish to sit down in a chair.

Use your stick until you feel that you can do without it.

Try to remain sleeping on your back. You may sleep on either side, but if you put your operated side uppermost place a pillow between your legs.

Take a shower at first or use aids for the bath as provided by the Occupational Therapy Department.

Use a shoe horn to put on shoes, and a stocking aid to put on tights.

Get into the car by putting your bottom in first and getting well back across the seat before swinging your legs in.

Avoid gardening. Do not kneel and avoid bending at the hip.

Avoid twisting on the affected leg.

It was explained to her that very occasionally a hip may dislocate and that the most vulnerable position in which this might happen occurs when the affected leg is bent at the hip and crossing over at the midline, i.e. sitting with your legs crossed.

Mrs Neilson's son came to collect her from the hospital. She was going to stay with him for a fortnight and then go to her daughter's for another two weeks. She left the ward with one week's supply of distalgesics, an outpatient appointment for six weeks' time and one stick. If she felt unwell she was to contact her G.P. If there were any activities she found that she was unable to do she was to contact the Occupational Therapy Department.

She left with a smile and a wave.

Six weeks later she returned for her follow-up appointment. By then she had discarded her stick, and the hip had healed well. She talked with delight of meeting her friends while walking Rebel again.

<table>
<tr><td>TEST
YOURSELF</td><td>1</td><td>Why did Mrs Neilson require a total hip replacement?</td></tr>
<tr><td></td><td>2</td><td>Was this the first line of treatment and why?</td></tr>
<tr><td></td><td>3</td><td>Which members of the orthopaedic team were involved in Mrs Neilson's care immediately prior to her operation and what is their function?</td></tr>
</table>

4 What observations should the nurses make concerning the operation on return to the ward?

5 What precautions should be taken to prevent damage to the affected limb?

6 How does Mrs Neilson's operation affect her activities of living?

7 What role does the physiotherapist play in her rehabilitation?

8 What role does the occupational therapist play in her rehabilitation?

FURTHER READING

ARTHRITIS AND RHEUMATISM COUNCIL. *Osteoarthrosis – A Handbook for Patients.* London: Arthritis and Rheumatism Council.

FARRELL, J. 1984. Orthopaedic Pain. What does it mean? *American Journal of Nursing* **84** (4), 466–8.

GOLDING, D. 1980. Osteoarthrosis. *The Practitioner* **224** (1), 19–24.

NOWOTNY, M. 1980. If Your Patient's Joints Hurt, the Reason May Be Osteoarthrosis. *Nursing (Horsham)* **10** (9), 39–41.

4 Mr Holmes, who sustains a Colles fracture

HISTORY

Mr Holmes, aged 80, lives in a small village in the heart of England. He and his wife have lived there for the last 50 years. Despite his age Mr Holmes is a very fit, healthy and active man. He is involved in local church affairs and running the social club, and is well known and liked by everyone in the village.

One frosty morning as Mr and Mrs Holmes were walking from their cottage to church, Mr Holmes suddenly slipped and fell onto the pavement. He reached out trying to save himself and fell onto his outstretched hand. Mrs Holmes was very anxious as she tried to help her husband to his feet. His right forearm was misshapen, and he was complaining of great pain.

Mr Walker, the church warden, was driving past when he saw Mrs Holmes struggling to get her husband to his feet. He helped them both into his car and took them to the Accident and Emergency (A&E) Department of the local hospital.

ADMISSION TO HOSPITAL

On their arrival in the department, they were welcomed by Linda, the accident and emergency nurse. She showed Mrs Holmes to the reception area for history taking and took Mr Holmes into the cubicle. She helped him to remove his overcoat, commencing from the uninjured side. Once she had helped him to remove his jacket, tie, shirt, and vest, Linda let Mr Holmes hold his right arm while she collected and applied a triangular sling. This supported his arm and made him more comfortable.

Before putting the sling on his arm Linda looked to see whether Mr Holmes was wearing a ring on his injured hand. (All rings must be removed. The injury will lead to oedema of the fingers and a ring would become a tight band and stop the circulation.) Looking at his right arm Linda could see that it was misshapen. She verified that she could feel a brachial pulse. She also noted that the hand was warm to the touch, that Mr Holmes could feel her touching his fingers and that he could wriggle his fingers. These observations are important to check for interference in circulation and for nerve damage. She informed the doctor that Mr Holmes was in a cubicle.

When the doctor examined Mr Holmes, he ordered an X-ray and informed him that he had sustained a fracture to his right arm known as a Colles fracture. They proceeded to the reception area to talk with Mrs Holmes.

What is a Colles fracture?

A Colles fracture is the name given to a fracture of the lower third of the radius with backward displacement of the fragment. This fragment is driven up and impacted into the proximal fragment. The ulna styloid can be intact or avulsed. This may produce a dinner fork deformity.

A Colles fracture

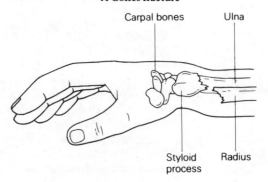

The doctor told them that the fracture must be straightened ('reduced'). This would be done there and then in the Accident and Emergency Department. The doctor asked Mr Holmes if he had had anything to eat or drink that morning. As he had eaten breakfast, he could not have a general anaesthetic because of the risk of inhaled vomit. Therefore the doctor explained to Mr Holmes that he would have a peripheral nerve block.

What is a peripheral nerve block?

This is a means by which a limb is anaesthetised, using intravenous analgesia. Other parts of the body are not anaesthetised.

The Anaesthetist puts a cannula needle into the back of the hand. The arm is then elevated to drain it of blood, and a double cuff is applied to the top of the arm. The top cuff (No. 1) is inflated above systolic pressure. The anaesthetist then injects an anaesthetic solution, e.g. marcaine 0.5%, via the cannula into the vein. It takes approximately 10 to 20 minutes for the solution to take effect. Then cuff No. 2 is also inflated to above systolic pressure and cuff No. 1 is then released. The cuff is therefore inflated on an anaesthetised skin and it is more comfortable for the patient. The procedure of reducing the fracture is then done by the doctor. When the procedure is complete the cuff is released slowly to allow the intravenous solution to pass gradually into the general circulation. During the procedure the arm looks very white and the patient must be warned about this. The nurse must observe the patient throughout the process. She must watch particularly closely when the cuff is being released. If too much anaesthetic is released suddenly into the circulation the patient may have a cardiac arrest.

Biers block

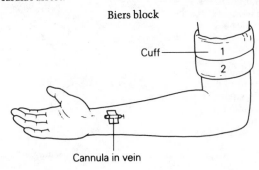

Cuff — 1
2

Cannula in vein

What is plaster of Paris (POP)?

Plaster of Paris is a material which looks like chalk and is embedded into a mesh bandage. When mixed with water, a chemical reaction takes place and the chalky material swells, giving off heat and setting rapidly. It then becomes a rock hard cement. Propriety brands used include Gypsona and Crystona.

How long does it take a POP to dry?

A small POP like this takes 3 to 4 minutes to set When first applied a POP feels hot to the patient.
12 to 24 hours later it feels cold and clammy.
24 to 48 hours later the POP feels normal to the patient and has the same body temperature.
All plasters take at least 48 hours to dry but it can take up to 72 hours depending on the weight and thickness of the plaster.

The doctor continued explaining to Mr Holmes that once reduced, the fracture would be immobilised in an incomplete plaster of Paris cast.

Plaster of Paris cast for a Colles fracture

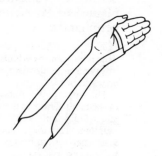

Incomplete POP held in place with bandage

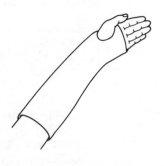

Complete POP

Initial stages

Mr Holmes signed his consent form as he knew this must be done but he expressed several fears to Linda. She listened to Mr Holmes ask, 'How much pain will I feel if I am not asleep? How long must I have the plaster on my arm and will my arm be as good as before the operation? Will they cut my arm open to do this operation?' Linda explained that the fracture is reduced by manipulation and that he would feel no pain as he would be given an anaesthetic, into his arm. She also explained that he would wear the plaster of Paris for six weeks and when it was removed he would then go to classes to exercise the wrist as it would be stiff. Mr Holmes talked to his wife about what the doctor and the nurse had told him and appeared calmer and less anxious. Mrs Holmes also seemed much happier. She collected her husband's belongings and waited in the reception area while he underwent the reduction of his fractured forearm. Linda observed Mr Holmes' condition throughout.

Immediately after application

1 Handle all wet POP's with the palm of the hand and support it in its entirety (a depression or crack in the POP cast can lead to a pressure sore). An inadvertent thumb pressure can cause a pressure sore.
2 Place a limb encased in a wet POP onto a pillow covered with plastic sheeting and a towel. Leave to the air to dry normally.
3 Note temperature, colour, swelling or loss of movement of the extremities (if there is any doubt about the circulation the plaster must be split).

4 Pain of the limb in a POP may indicate ischaemia or gangrene of the extremities.

A split plaster of Paris

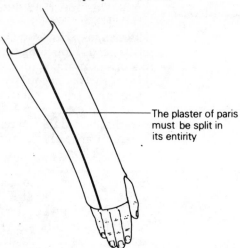

The plaster of paris must be split in its entirity

Observation of Mr Holmes' right arm immobilised in a plaster of Paris

1 Place the limb on a plastic covered pillow.
2 Observe the fingers for warmth, colour – pink – and quick circulatory return, sensation to touch, movement – opposition of thumb to all fingers – and swelling of fingers.
3 Check that movement of flexion and extension is possible at the elbow.
4 Check the brachial pulse on his right arm as it will be impossible to take the radial pulse and compare that pulse with the one on the left arm; both should be the same.
5 On finding any of the above, the nurse learner would of course report this to the person in charge of the ward.

The limb may become blue and cold to the touch if the blood vessels are compressed.

Numbness, tingling, pins and needles, lack of sensation and inability to move the extremities indicates compression of a nerve.

Any pressure or internal roughness of the POP cast may cause plaster sores.

Evaluation   Mr Holmes was able to move all his fingers, which felt warm to touch. His fingers were pink and though they were swollen he was able to feel them all.

Planning discharge

Mr Holmes remained a little drowsy because of the anaesthetic but was very relieved it was all over. Mrs Holmes came into the cubicle and sat with him until the doctor said he could go home. The doctor asked for another X-ray of Mr Holmes' arm now that he was in the POP. The X-ray showed that the fracture was in good alignment. Linda discussed Mr Holmes' care with his wife. Mrs Holmes is 80 years of age and Linda wanted to make sure as far as she could that she would be able to cope with her husband that night before he returned to the fracture clinic the next day to have his plaster of Paris cast completed.

N.B.   No patient is allowed to leave the hospital until all staff are satisfied that the circulation to the extremity of the limb is unimpaired.

Before his discharge Mr and Mrs Holmes are given both verbal and written instructions. Written instructions are very important as few people are able in these kinds of stressful situations to remember verbal information.

Instructions given to Mr Holmes

Mr Holmes is to return to the fracture clinic on the following morning for the completion of his POP cast. Linda ascertains that the church warden will be able to bring him in

Keep the POP cast dry at all times

Move all the joints not encased in POP

If there is any swelling, elevate the arm by putting it on pillows or in a sling

Mr Holmes must return to the department immediately if:

He is unable to move or feel his fingers

The POP feels too tight or his fingers are swollen and blue

The POP cast cracks

He feels any burning or itching below the POP causing pain

The nurse placed the arm in the POP cast in a triangular sling as it will feel heavy. This position also helps to reduce swelling.

Mr Holmes was given some paracetamol tablets to be taken 4 to 6 hourly for the pain. Mr Walker, who had been waiting in reception, took Mr and Mrs Holmes home.

On his return the next morning he told Linda that he had not had a very good night's sleep as every time he turned in bed he forgot about his arm and hit himself with the cast. He was also surprised to find that the cast was so heavy. Once the cast was complete, he was given the same instructions again.

The doctor sent him to see Jane, the occupational therapist, to assess the activity of his fingers. He was also sent to see Mary, the physiotherapist, to be instructed in arm exercises as it is very easy for elderly patients not to move the whole arm and end up with a stiff shoulder.

Complications of plaster casts:

1 Blood vessels may become compressed and the limb appear:

Blue

Swollen

Cold to the touch

2 Compression of the nerve supply. The patient complains of:
   Numbness
   A tingling sensation
   Pins and needles
   Inability to move the extremities
3 Too tight a plaster can cause the POP to rub the skin and plaster sores may arise. Loose material, e.g. coins or food, put into the plaster (perhaps to scratch the skin underneath) can also cause plaster sores.
4 Muscles under the cast can become atrophied; therefore static muscle contraction must be encouraged.
5 Joints under the POP casts become stiff.
6 Dried skin under a plaster can cause irritation.

NURSING CARE

Evaluation and rehabilitation

After six weeks in a plaster cast, Mr Holmes returned to the Outpatient Department. He had had a very uneventful time at home with his plaster of Paris cast.

He found that washing was very difficult as he was right handed. Mrs Holmes had to help him. He said that though he placed a plastic bag over his arm he was afraid of getting the plaster wet.

Combing his hair was difficult as the plaster did not bend. Using his left hand he nearly gave himself a black eye because his movements were so un-coordinated.

Mr Holmes said he was surprised how heavy his arm felt at first and how turning over in bed he had hurt himself and Mrs Holmes. No damage was done and they laughed. Mr Holmes, winking at Linda, mentioned that he soon learnt how to use his left arm to drink his pint of beer.

An X-ray of his arm in POP was taken. It showed union of his fracture and the doctor asked for the POP to be removed. After removal Mr Holmes was a bit shocked to see that his arm looked so skinny because of muscle wasting and scaly due to dry skin. Linda applied oil to the skin.

She explained to them that the skin was dry because it had been encased in the POP and they need only apply some oil until the scales flaked off. Mr Holmes found that he was unable to move his wrist. He was horrified. Linda said that this was normal because of the length of time his arm had been in a plaster cast. She gave him a sling and warned him that his fingers would swell for the first few days. She then made arrangements for him to see the community physiotherapist.

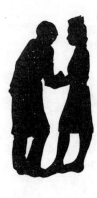

The community physiotherapist, Sarah Day, welcomed Mr Holmes and mentioned that she held classes three times a week at the health centre near his home. These classes will help Mr Holmes' wrist regain movement. Mr Holmes enjoyed these classes as he was joined by others who had sustained similar injuries. Sarah taught them to do their exercises to music. They also used therapeutic wax, doing twisting movements to encourage supination and pronation.

Then in the afternoon three times a week Mr Holmes also visited the Occupational Therapy Department at the hospital. Here he was engaged in using the printing press. This he found fun, helpful to his wrist and satisfying also, because he was doing printing work for a church function. This regime continued for four weeks.

The functional activity with the printing press helps to reduce oedema in wrist and hand and also strengthens and increases the range of movements of the joints of the hand.

In all it took Mr Holmes 10 weeks from the date of his injury before he was able to fully use his wrist. However he still says that he knows when it is going to rain because of the dull ache he gets in his wrist. Mrs Holmes tells Linda that it is true; when he complains, it rains.

1 What observations did the nurse make prior to Mr Holmes' reduction of his fracture?

2 Why is a Biers Block used?

3 What observations did the nurse make concerning the care of the forearm in plaster of Paris?

4 What instructions would you give to Mr Holmes concerning his plaster of Paris?

5 How did having his arm in a plaster of Paris cast affect Mr Holmes' activities of living?

6 What did Mr Holmes gain from attending occupational therapy and physiotherapy?

FURTHER
READING

BETTS-SYMONDS, G. W. 1984. *Fracture Care and Management for Students.* London: Macmillan Publishers Limited.
Post Basic Nursing Procedures – 10 – Plaster Casts 1. 1982. *Nursing Mirror* **154** (25), 28–9.
Post Basic Nursing Procedures – 11 – Plaster Casts 2. 1982. *Nursing Mirror* **154** (26), 28–9.
SMITH AND NEPHEW. *Plaster of Paris Technique: A Handbook for Students.* London.

5 Mrs Carter, a grandmother with a fractured neck of femur

Mrs Carter, aged 82 years, lives in a small cottage on her son's farm. She likes to live on her own, but enjoys the daily visit from her grandchildren, Christine, aged 8, and Stephen, aged 10. They always pass her house on their way to school, ringing the bells on their bicycles as they go.

On the way back from school they stop and chat with their grandmother before going riding. Mrs Carter enjoys watching her grandchildren ride in the evenings. During the day she enjoys watching the horses in the field next to her cottage.

One evening after the children had gone, she went to check the paddock gate to make sure that the horses were well secured for the night. Turning to go back to her cottage she stumbled and fell heavily to the ground.

She tried to get up but was unable to stand. In fact she found that she was in great pain and was unable to lift her left leg.

Her son had been looking for his mother at her cottage, and hearing her cries for help, he found her on the ground by the paddock gate.

He ran to the cottage to call for an ambulance. Before returning to his mother, he grabbed a shawl to keep her warm and stayed talking with her until the ambulance arrived.

ADMISSION TO THE HOSPITAL

On arrival at the hospital Mrs Carter was examined in the A&E Department by the Doc-

48

tor. By listening to her story and looking at her leg he quickly came to a diagnosis. Her left leg was lying externally rotated and there was obvious shortening. She was unable to move her leg and was in great pain. The Doctor ordered an X-ray of her hip and told Mrs Carter and her son that she had sustained an intertrochanteric fracture of the femoral neck and must be admitted urgently.

An intertrochanteric fracture of the femur is a break in the continuity of bone between the trochanters of the femur (No. 4).

What is an intertrochanteric fracture of the femur?
Fractures of the femur can be divided into two main types:
1 Intracapsular
2 Extracapsular

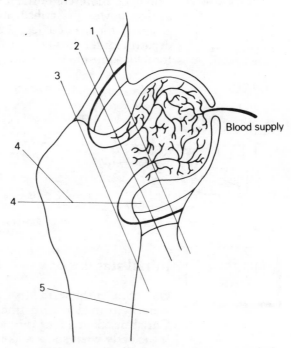

Blood supply

Fractures through the neck of femur are intracapsular, e.g. 1 (subcapital) and 2 (transcervical). Fractures through the trochanters of the femur are extracapsular, e.g. 3 (pertrochanteric), 4 (intertrochanteric) and 5 (subtrochanteric).

49

The femoral head has a good blood supply which is essential for bone healing. However the main source of blood is from the capsular vessels high in the femoral neck; if these are damaged the femoral head may receive less blood, causing it to die (*avascular necrosis*). The treatment of choice is to replace the femoral head with a stem prosthesis. However, if the fracture is extracapsular, there is less likelihood of damaging all the blood supply and the treatment of choice is then to pin and plate the fracture.

Traction is a pull along a line. The resistance to this pull is the patient and is known as counter traction. Skin traction involves a strap which may be adhesive or non-adhesive and is applied to the leg. The distal end is attached by a cord to a weight via a pulley system

The doctor explained that she would require an operation. As Mrs Carter had eaten only a few hours ago, she would have to have her operation the following morning. So that she would be more comfortable for the evening analgesia was prescribed and skin traction arranged for her left leg. Before leaving the department for the Orthopaedic ward the doctor took some blood tests.

Skin traction

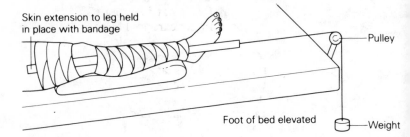

Skin extension to leg held in place with bandage

Pulley

Foot of bed elevated

Weight

NURSING CARE

Initial stages

On arrival at the ward Mrs Carter and her son were welcomed by Christine, the ward nurse. Christine spent a long time with her explaining exactly what she was doing. She was very careful not to cause Mrs Carter any extra pain when moving her from the trolley and placing her on the bed. Mrs Carter appeared pale, in severe pain, with a bruised and swollen left hip. Christine explained that the non-adhesive skin extensions would be bandaged to her leg and that this would reduce muscle spasm and prevent any further damage overnight. This type of skin extension was used as it would be removed the following morning. Christine collected as much information from her patient about her fears, likes and dislikes, noting that Mrs Carter was not fat. She took baseline observations. Mrs Carter told Christine that she had the same name as her granddaughter.

<table>
<tr><td>

**CARE
PLAN**

</td><td>

for Mrs Carter pre-operatively

</td></tr>
</table>

Potential problem She is probably confused due to the shock of the injury and must be reoriented in time and place.
Nursing care and rationale Explain all procedures in simple terms before they happen. Allow her son to stay with her until he feels reassured about her well-being. Remind her where she is and what is going to occur. Involve her son in her care so that he may repeat it to her later.

Establishing communication with her is important to differentiate between her being emotionally upset due to the trauma or disorientated.
Evaluation Mrs Carter did not become confused pre-operatively. Her son stayed with her until 11 o'clock that evening, only leaving after receiving instructions of what she required from home and where to find it.

Potential problem Inactivity and pain are conducive to shallow breathing. It is important to encourage deep breathing to keep the lung fields clear, or infection may occur.
Nursing care and rationale The physiotherapist should visit to instruct her in deep breathing exercises.

Also the anaesthetist will see her before her operation and take a chest X-ray.

Lung expansion and clearance are essential as otherwise retained secretions collect in the alveolar sacs and may become infected.

Evaluation Mrs Carter was very apprehensive but found the breathing exercises easy to do. She did not like having her chest X-rayed because of the pain in her leg whenever she was moved.

Actual problem Enforced bedrest is necessary because of the skin traction to immobilise the leg by reducing muscle spasm. It has many potential complications.

Nursing care and rationale Observe the hip area for swelling. The skin extensions must remain in place. If the bandage is wrinkled or if it has slipped and is around the ankle it must be reapplied. Ensure that the cord is taut, the pulley is running freely and the weight is hanging free. It is essential that the traction equipment is in good working order. Make sure that the foot of the bed is elevated and therefore that the traction and counter traction are being maintained. A divided bed is used to allow room for knee exercises. A bed cradle helps to keep the weight of the bedclothes off the leg. Watch the leg and foot closely; too tight bandages cause constriction of blood vessels.

Evaluation Mrs Carter said the pull on her leg stopped the grating sound and her leg stopped shaking. She became very anxious if someone walked close to the hanging weight as hitting it hurt her leg.

Potential problem Her prominent areas must be prevented from developing pressure sores due to being on traction.

Nursing care and rationale Look at all the pressure areas and assess the patient's condition using the Norton scale. Move her two-hourly from side to side. Use sheepskin under the heels or sheepskin bootees. Clear the drawsheet of crumbs and straighten any wrinkling of the sheet.

Turning the patient two-hourly prevents pressure sores (Norton *et al.*, 1962). There must be a strict enforcement of the turning regime for it to be effective (Berecek, 1975).

Evaluation Mrs Carter complained of soreness at the base of her spine. Being a thin lady she was moved two-hourly from side to side, and pillows were used to keep her off her sacral area. Using the Norton scale she scored 13. She sat up for her meals and preferred only two pillows at night.

Potential problem Urinary difficulties because of the unnatural position for voiding urine may lead to urinary stasis and thence to infection.

Nursing care and rationale Offer her a slipper bedpan regularly. Obtain a routine urine ward sample and test it before she goes for operation. Encourage her to drink 1 litre before her operation, that is until she must be nil by mouth.

Many elderly patients limit their fluid intake in order not to need to use the bedpan. This causes the patient to become dehydrated, leading to reduced urinary output and urinary stasis.

Evaluation Mrs Carter was at first reluctant to drink but when the nurse explained the reason, she drank as much as she could – 600 ml from 10 o'clock until 2 o'clock in the morning. She voided 350 ml of urine and no abnormality was observed on ward testing.

Actual problem There is pain due to the fracture which must be relieved.

Nursing care Administer dextroproposyphene and paracetamol as prescribed by the doctor (distalgesic tablets given 4–6 hourly as necessary). Premedication is due at 8 o'clock in the morning.

Good pain relief is essential. Pain will limit movement and invite the complications attendent on bedrest and surgery (Bloore, 1979).

Mrs Carter did not suffer any other problems. She remained on skin traction for 10 hours before her operation. She slept fitfully on the ward surrounded by so many patients as she was used to the quiet of her cottage. However, she appeared calm before her operation.

Research about pressure sores

The use of alcohol, methylated spirit and other astringents are harmful to the skin (Torrance, 1983). The use of witch hazel makes the tissues more vulnerable to pressure sores (Norton *et al.*, 1962). Torrance (1983) suggests that there is doubtful value in the use of creams, sprays and lotions. Vigorous rubbing or massage is harmful (Dyson, 1978).

Methods of preventing pressure sores:
1 Move the patient regularly (Norton *et al.*, 1962).
2 Observe the skin and keep it clean.
3 Use of aids, e.g. sheepskins, ripple mattress (large cell only), bed cradle. The nurse must understand how to use these aids so that they are effective.

The Norton Scale or the pressure sore risk assessment form (*Report of Investigation in Geriatric Nursing Problems in Hospital*, Norton *et al.*, 1962)

General Condition	Mental state	Activity	Mobility	Incontinence
4 good	4 alert	4 ambulant	4 full	4 not
3 fair	3 apathetic	3 walks help	3 limited	3 occasional
2 poor	2 confused	2 chairbound	2 very limited	2 usually urine
1 very bad	1 stupor	1 bed	1 immobile	1 doubly

A high score of 20 indicates good general health, mentally alert, active, fully mobile and continent. A score of 14 or below = at risk.

Before Mrs Carter's operation Christine carried out a pre-operative check list (p. 3). Mrs Carter was taken to the operating theatre in her bed. Christine told her that she will awaken initially in the recovery room next to the operating theatre and only when fully awake will she return to the ward. The doctor, having explained to Mrs Carter that she will have a plate and nail to hold the fracture together and a drain from her hip, also tells her that she will be up in a chair the next day, which is one of the great benefits of this operation. Usually a fractured femur would require about three months of bed rest to heal. Christine added that she will be given some analgesia before getting up, and Mrs Carter looked a little easier.

Mrs Carter returned to the ward, following a fixation with a plate and nail fixation.

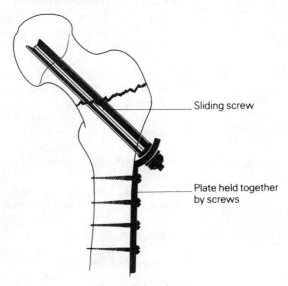

Nail and plate fixation

CARE PLAN

for Mrs Carter postoperatively

Potential problem She may be unable to maintain an adequate fluid balance and must not be allowed to dehydrate.
Nursing care and rationale Monitor her IV infusion line. Observe the needle site on the arm for redness and swelling of the tissues. Any redness at the infusion site may indicate a phlebitis and swelling may mean that the

needle is in the tissues instead of in the vein.

Encourage Mrs Carter to take liquids as soon as bowel sounds are heard. Record all intake on the fluid balance chart. Anaesthesia causes the digestive tract to stop working. It is important to ensure that it has started working again before the patient is allowed to eat or drink as otherwise vomiting will occur. This condition is known as a paralytic ileus.

Evaluation The doctor discontinued Mrs Carter's IV infusion as soon as bowel sounds were heard. She started off just drinking water and then when this was well tolerated she could have whatever she wanted.

Potential problem Many people, but particularly the elderly, become confused after surgery. This usually wears off with time, but relatives must be warned of this effect. It is important to maintain normal communication with the patients, even if this involves constantly repeating where they are and what you are doing.

Nursing care and rationale Explain to Mrs Carter that she has had her operation, and all procedures that you are carrying out as you are performing them.

The elderly become confused for several reasons: if they are removed from their familiar surroundings into a place that they do not know, if there is an underlying disease, or infection or fever or shock. They may be haemorrhaging and the loss of blood may cause an electrolyte imbalance, which will affect their mental state.

Evaluation Mrs Carter became disorientated. She did not know where she was, though the nurses told her each time they spent some time with her. She attempted to get out of bed because she said that the pigeons were coming to get her. Unfortunately there was no low bed on the ward so the nurses had to put up the cot sides. The family were extremely disturbed by this and were reassured and supported by Jenny Bell, the ward sister, and her nurses. Mrs Carter remained confused and disorientated for one week and gradually improved over the next three weeks.

Potential problem Pressure sores may develop as a result of the enforced bed rest.

Nursing care and rationale Check all pressure points when helping her with washing. When she is in bed, turn her 2–4-hourly. Place a pillow between her legs as this helps to prevent strain on the hip. She can be turned on either side.

Encourage Mrs Carter to use her monkey pole to help move herself around and change position.

Evaluation Mrs Carter's heels looked red but no sore developed.

Potential problem Urinary tract infection is a possible complication of enforced bed rest. Active steps are required to prevent it, bearing in mind its causes.

Nursing care and rationale Encourage Mrs Carter to drink at least 1500 ml of fluid per day, of whatever kind she prefers (usually hot chocolate).

Offer bedpans regularly. When Mrs Carter is out of bed, offer her a commode. Check the colour and amount of urine, and record this on a fluid intake/output chart.

Evaluation Mrs Carter was reluctant to drink at first but when Christine asked her to help fill in her fluid balance chart and explained the reasons for this, her intake improved.

Potential problem Joint stiffness and contractions may result due to her inactivity and this must be prevented to maintain maximum mobility of her limbs.

Nursing care and rationale She should be

seen by the physiotherapist daily. Encourage her to move her ankles (see p. 11). She will probably have a check X-ray 48 hours after the operation. Remind her to sit out on a chair rather than stay in bed. When moving Mrs Carter from the bed to a chair always move the left (damaged) leg first and therefore get her out on the left side of bed. This ensures that there will be no dragging of her injured leg and she can move the uninjured leg easily.

Evaluation Mrs Carter's X-ray showed that her fracture was being held in a good position. She did not like sitting in the chair because the wound was painful. Christine discussed with Mary, the physiotherapist, when it was best to sit her in the chair for her exercises so that she could arrange to give her some analgesia half an hour before moving her.

Potential problem Deep vein thrombosis may arise as a complication of bed rest and lack of movement of the legs. It is important to prevent the venous stasis which leads to this.

Nursing care and rationale She should wear elastic stockings on both legs to encourage venous return. Remove them each day and check the skin for abrasions.

Evaluation Mrs Carter did not suffer a deep vein thrombosis but her left leg did look swollen. Christine kept that leg elevated and encouraged her to do her ankle movements 5 times every hour.

NURSING
CARE

Rehabilitation

Mrs Carter's recovery was slow. She was very confused and disorientated during the first week of hospitalisation. Christine spent many hours explaining to her where she was and what was happening to her. The family needed much support and reassurance during this time as it was very disturbing for them to see her so confused. In order to help Mrs Carter with her confusion, family photographs were brought in from her home so that she would have something familiar near her.

Jane, the occupational therapist, came to see Mrs Carter to assess what she could do for herself when she went home. She suggested that Mrs Carter should visit the department to be assessed for how well she could cope with dressing and making a cup of tea. After this visit Mrs Carter wore her own clothes; she had a nap after lunch and seemed much brighter than before.

Mrs Carter was able to put full weight on her left leg but had more confidence walking if she had her sticks. She always complained of pain in her hip, however, and she found that taking her analgesia before seeing Jane and Mary helped considerably. Her hip sutures were removed on the fourteenth day.

Planning discharge

It was six weeks before Mrs Carter recovered enough to go home. She still needed a great deal of support and before she was discharged it was arranged that she should come to the hospital three times a week for functional assessment in the Occupational Therapy Department. Mrs Carter would also go to the Physiotherapy Department by ambulance for hydrotherapy treatment. Christine ascertained that she was not afraid of pools and indeed had been quite fond of swimming in her youth. This therapy appeared to help her walking.

Mrs Carter insisted on going home. Her family popped in each day to make sure that she was all right and brought her meals. The district nurse dropped by to see that she was coping and also to find out whether the family were managing.

After three weeks as an outpatient Mrs Carter did not require any more physiotherapy and she was looking after herself again. On the 12th week she came to see the nurses on the ward before visiting the doctor. She was cheerful on arrival but she seemed to have aged.

TEST YOURSELF

1 Why was Mrs Carter's limb externally rotated?

2 What was Mrs Carter and her son told about her fracture prior to her operation?

3 Why did the nurse plan for potential problems prior to Mrs Carter's operation and why were these problems important?

4 What is the 'Norton Scale' and why is it used?

5 How did Mrs Carter's care differ postoperatively from pre-operatively?

6 What problems did Mrs Carter and her family experience?

7 How many people were involved in Mrs Carter's rehabilitation and how did they help her?

8 How was Mrs Carter's family helped to cope with her postoperative confusion and disorientation?

FURTHER READING

BERECEK, K. H. 1975. Treatment of Decubitus Ulcers. *Nursing Clinics of North America* 10 (1), 171–210.

BLOORE, J. R. P. 1979. Nursing Surgical Patients in Acute Pain. *Nursing (Oxford)* 1 (1), 37–44.

DYSON, R. 1978. Bedsores – The Injuries Hospital Staff Inflict on Patients. *Nursing Mirror* 146 (24), 30–32.

GODINA, E. 1981. Make a Break, Femur Fracture in an Elderly Patient. *Nursing Mirror* **153** (13), 32–34.
HANNA, A. 1982. Make a Break. *Nursing Mirror* **155** (15), 59–61.
NORTON, D. *et al.* 1962. *Investigation of Geriatric Nursing Problems in Hospital.* London NCCOP. Re-issued (1975) Edinburgh: Churchill Livingstone.
TORRANCE, C. 1983. *Pressure Sores, Aetiology, Treatment and Prevention.* London: Croom Helm.

6

Mr Walters, who suffers from rheumatoid arthritis

HISTORY

Rheumatoid arthritis is a chronic inflammatory disease affecting the synovial membrane within a joint. The disease is progressive and from time to time the patient suffers acute exacerbations (flare-ups) and then remissions. This condition is more common in women than in men. The disease manifests itself between the ages of 20 and 50.

Which joints are affected? It is more common in the hands, wrists, feet, knees, shoulders and neck. However any synovial joint may be involved and it is usually symmetrical in distribution, e.g. both knees or both wrists.

Mr Walters is 60 years of age. He lives with his wife in a third floor council flat in a busy town. He and his wife have three grown-up children who have all left home. His two daughters are married and live in Europe. His married son, a policeman, lives nearby.

Mr Walters' hobbies include gardening (his son has an allotment), watching cricket and going to the local pub for a pint and a chat.

He has suffered from rheumatoid arthritis for 23 years.

What occurs in the joint?
In Figure (b) plasma cells and lymphocytes infiltrate the joint causing inflammation of the synovial membrane. The synovial membrane produces more synovial fluid and the joint becomes swollen and painful.

This chronic inflammation of the synovial membrane leads to finger-like projections from the membrane into the synovial fluid which are known as pannus. The now deformed synovial membrane produces enzymes and the rheumatoid factor that wears away the articular cartilage.

The joint becomes deformed and degenerative changes in the articular cartilage may eventually lead to osteoarthrosis (see Chapter 3). The disease does not contain itself just to the joint; it can wear away tendons, causing them to snap, as well as causing inflammation in other tissues, e.g. lung, heart and eyes.

What is the cause of rheumatoid arthritis?
The direct cause of rheumatoid arthritis is unknown. The main theories which have been put forward to explain it are:

    Infection, e.g. virus
    Heredity
    Allergy and stress
    Auto-immune disease

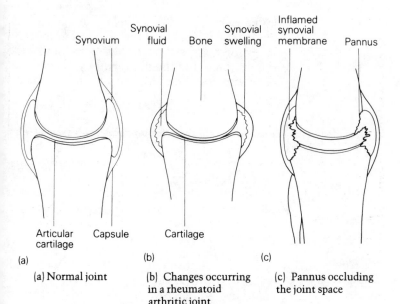

(a) Normal joint	(b) Changes occurring in a rheumatoid arthritic joint	(c) Pannus occluding the joint space

The last is currently the most favoured. It is believed that there is some alteration in a body's cell make-up either due to a virus or to the inability to recognise its own cells. This causes the immune system to treat one of the body's own cells as 'foreign'. The body's defence mechanism then forms antibodies to fight the 'foreign' cells. One of these antibodies is known as the rheumatoid factor and is found in the blood of patients suffering from rheumatoid arthritis. These antibodies destroy the surrounding tissue.

Signs and symptoms:
A person may complain of any of the following symptoms to their doctor:
    Feeling unwell over many months
    Pain and stiffness of joints especially in the morning
    Swelling of the joint
    Tiredness and lethargy
    Loss of weight
    Anaemia
    Muscle pain and muscle wasting
    Anxiety and depression

Mr Walters has over the past few years had problems with his shoulders, hands and feet. Lately he can hardly walk because of the pain in his right knee; he can bend it to 90 degrees but it is stiff. He has taken anti-inflammatory drugs for years, although these were not effective in removing the pain. Finally his general practitioner referred him to a hospital consultant.

Rheumatoid arthritis affecting shoulders, hands and feet

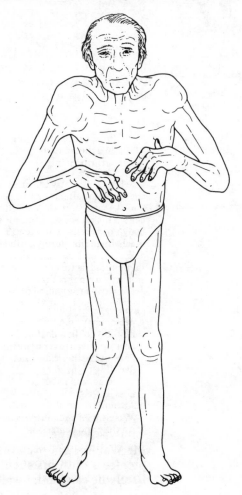

Mr Walters received a letter requesting him to visit the consultant a few weeks later. After examination the consultant said that his right knee joint was badly damaged and that he would require a knee replacement.

Six weeks later Mr Walters received a letter from the hospital informing him that there was a bed vacant on the following Monday.

ADMISSION
TO THE
WARD

Mr Walters arrived at the ward where he was welcomed by Christine. She was expecting him and showed him to his bed. She explained how the call bell system, radio and lights worked and where to find the toilet and bathroom. She then introduced him to the five other patients in his bay.

NURSING
CARE

Initial stages

Christine then told him that his operation would be in two days' time as he would undergo several investigations prior to it. He would be visited by the doctor and the anaesthetist who would both examine him.

Several tests would be ordered including a chest X-ray, blood tests and an ECG to ensure that he was fit for the operation.

Christine chatted to Mr Walters while taking his temperature, pulse, respirations and wrote up a nursing history. These observations are used as a base line when assessing Mr Walter's condition in the future. She said that if there was anything he wanted to know or discuss, she would try to help.

He was a little apprehensive about his operation. He mentioned that his wife was not in good health and would not be able to visit him frequently, but would telephone the ward. Christine said that there was a trolley telephone which he could use, all he had to do was ask.

Christine explained that Mr Walters would not wake up in the ward, but in the recovery room and that as soon as his observations were stable he would return to the ward. She also told him that his leg would be covered by a large bandage, and partially encased in plaster of Paris. He would also have one or two vacuum drains from his knee wound for about twenty-four hours to help prevent haematoma formation.

CARE PLAN

for Mr Walters pre-operatively

Actual problem Pain from the rheumatoid arthritis and his damaged knee leads to immobility and must be relieved or controlled to maintain comfort.

Nursing care and rationale As Mr Walters is in constant pain he is also at risk of developing pressure sores. Turn him two-hourly and place sheepskin bootees on his heels. Place a pillow between his legs when he is on his side as correct positioning of the body puts less strain on the muscles and joints and also relieves the pain.

Regular analgesia is important to control pain (see p. 4). Use a bed cradle to keep the weight of the bed clothes off his legs and feet. Encourage him to move within his limitations to keep his independence.

Evaluation Mr Walters was unable to lift himself up due to pain in his hands and shoulders and could not use the 'monkey pole' for assistance. He was able to move in bed by rolling from side to side.

He remained in some pain but he said that he was used to this and it was a way of life.

Potential problem The deformity of hands

and inability to move without pain make it very difficult for Mr Walters to maintain his personal hygiene.

Nursing care and rationale Mr Walters prefers to be lifted into the bath using the hoist if his joints are very stiff on wakening. If he is in pain he would rather have a bed bath. Heat decreases pain and relaxes muscles thus assisting the patient to move more easily.

At these times inspect pressure points for signs of developing pressure sores (see Chapter 2).

Evaluation Mr Walters found having a hot bath very helpful as it eased his pains throughout the day.

Potential problem He is anxious about the forthcoming operation.

Nursing care and rationale Talk to Mr Walters about all the procedures before his operation and involve his relatives so that they know what will be happening. Also explain to them what will happen after his operation, e.g. that his temperature, pulse and respirations will be taken every four hours. Ensure that they understand as in this rather stressful situation people will not always remember much of what you tell them. Information helps the patient to understand and accept what is happening. Also something which you deal with daily and take for granted may seem very alarming to the patient who is actually having the operation.

Evaluation Mr Walters talked to the nurses, the physiotherapist and the doctor about his operation and, although anxious, felt more at ease.

Mr Walters was first on the theatre list that morning. His joints were very stiff so the night staff helped him with his bed bath. Christine carried out the pre-operation checklist. All was well. She accompanied him to the operating theatre and stayed with him until he was anaesthetised.

Mr Walters had a total knee replacement and returned to the ward from the recovery room fully awake.

for Mr Walters postoperatively

Potential problem The wound may haemorrhage through the plaster of Paris.

Nursing care and rationale Inspect the two vacuum drains regularly.

Keep watch on Mr Walter's wound to note any bleeding through the plaster of Paris and bandage. Draw a circle round any oozing and mark with date and time. This will enable you to determine, roughly, the rate and amount of bleeding occurring and whether any corrective actions should be taken.

Cover the pillow with a plastic cover and a towel until the POP is dry as the towel will absorb the moisture. Elevate the foot of bed. Examine the patient's foot for warmth, colour, sensation, movement and pedal pulse, as well as observing for excessive swelling. Any of the above signs shows an impaired circulation and the doctor must be notified immediately.

Evaluation There was no bleeding into the plaster of Paris, and the vacuum drains were removed after 48 hours. His leg was elevated on a pillow and the foot of the bed was tilted. His toes were swollen for the first 48 hours but colour, sensation, warmth and movement of the toes were satisfactory.

After 14 days the plaster was cut in half (bi-valved) and the sutures were removed. The back half of the old plaster cast (back slab) was retained and used as a splint when Mr Walters was walking or asleep.

Actual problem He will be unable to some degree to maintain his personal hygiene needs.

Nursing care and rationale   Help Mr Walters with his bed bath, but encourage him to do as much as possible as this will aid his return to independence. As he gets better, wheel him out to the basin in the bathroom with his leg elevated on a leg piece.

Evaluation   Mr Walters found that when his intravenous infusion line was removed from his right arm he was able to manage his personal hygiene as before. He preferred washing at the sink if the nurse could find a wheelchair with a leg piece to keep his foot elevated.

Potential problem   He may suffer from urinary retention and constipation and it is important to maintain normal bowel and bladder action.

Nursing care and rationale   Offer Mr Walters a urinal at frequent intervals. To ensure a good diuresis persuade him to drink at least 3 litres per day. Immobility can cause retention of urine.

Encourage him to eat high fibre foods as anaesthetics cause slowing of the digestive tract and immobility can lead to constipation.

Evaluation   Mr Walters found that he was unable to pass urine for 10 hours after his operation. Christine turned on the water taps so that he could hear the sound of running water. This proved to be the solution to the problem.

Potential problem   There is a risk of pressure sores developing on his heels, sacrum, elbows and under the plaster of Paris.

Nursing care and rationale   Change Mr Walters' position every two hours, scrutinising the pressure points carefully and reporting any change in the condition of his skin. Verify that the edges of the plaster do not rub the skin and cause redness. Report any complaints of soreness, a burning sensation or itchiness under the POP as any of the above may indicate a plaster sore (see pressure sores, Chapter 4).

Evaluation Mr Walters complained of sore elbows from moving himself around his bed. He found the application of some dermalex lotion soothing. The back half of the plaster of Paris cast did not cause him any difficulties.

Potential problem Wound infection is always a possible complication of surgery and every step must be taken to prevent it.

Nursing care and rationale Inspect the dressing for oozing and haemorrhaging. Examine the wound for any swelling and pain. Take his temperature every four hours; if it is above 37.5°C inform the nurse in charge immediately. There is often a rise in temperature during the first 48 hours due to the inflammatory response. If the temperature is elevated after 96 hours then a wound infection is suspected.

Evaluation Mr Walters' temperature was elevated to 38.0°C during the first 48 hours, then remained at 36.8°C for the rest of his stay in hospital.

Potential problem Deep vein thrombosis due to venous stasis may occur and it is important to maintain circulation and muscle tone.

Nursing care and rationale Mr Walters will wear an anti-embolitic stocking on the unaffected leg. Report any tenderness in the calf or groin, as any compression of the veins causes venous stasis which may lead to a blood clot formation (thrombus). Should this thrombus become dislodged it may block the vein, causing pain, tenderness and ischaemia. Muscle action prevents venous stasis and increases blood flow. Encourage Mr Walters to do his ankle movements (see p. 11).

Evaluation Mr Walters had no calf pain. He sat out in an armchair on the second day after the operation.

Potential problem   Wasting of the quadriceps muscles may occur and leads to instability of the knee joint.

Nursing care and rationale   Quadriceps exercises for both legs were demonstrated by Mary, the physiotherapist and Mr Walters must be encouraged to do them often. He should try out his exercises on his unaffected leg first and then do these exercises on his operated leg.

Lie in bed with both legs straight out in front
Bring the foot up to right angles (90°)
Tighten thigh muscle (quadriceps) by pushing the back of the thigh into the bed
Once this has been accomplished lift the leg off the bed (straight leg raising)

Evaluation   Mr Walters was able to do his quadriceps exercises by the fifth day after the operation. Once this was accomplished he could then do a 'straight leg raise' exercise.

NURSING CARE

Rehabilitation

Mr Walters' recovery was uneventful. He had days when he was in pain from his condition, and this was controlled by analgesia and anti-inflammatory drugs.

Two weeks after the operation, when the POP was bi-valved, Mr Walters' wound was found to be well healed. Every week day morning he was taken in his wheelchair to the hydrotherapy pool. Here with the help of Mary he did exercises under water. Mary's aim was to get 90° of flexion at the knee joint so that she could teach him to walk again. He still carried on doing his leg exercises on the ward. He found that on some days he did well and on others the pain and stiffness in his shoulders and hands was so severe that he felt he would never achieve his goal of walking independently again. He commenced walking with a rollator on the 14th day after his operation.

His wife came to see him whenever their son could bring her in the car. However Mr Walters spoke to her daily on the telephone.

He persevered with his exercises and walking, encouraged and praised by all involved in his care. After three weeks he was delighted to find that he could bend his knee.

He was assessed by Jane, the occupational therapist, in the department to see what he could do for himself. Jane assessed his activities of living; he practised dressing, transferring from the bed to a chair and making himself a cup of tea.

NURSING CARE

Planning discharge

Before he went home Mary verified that Mr Walters understood the exercises that he could do at home. She also made sure that he could negotiate the stairs in his house. Christine explained that she had ordered one week's supply of drugs that would control his pain and his rheumatoid arthritic condition. However he would have to go to his G.P. for repeat prescriptions. An outpatients' appointment was arranged for six weeks' time.

TEST YOURSELF

1 What do you understand by the term rheumatoid arthritis?

2 What information was Mr Walters given prior to his operation?

3 What observations should the nurse make concerning the operation on his return to the ward?

4 What precautions should be taken to prevent any damage to the affected limb?

5 How does Mr Walters knee replacement affect his activities of living?

6 What role do other members of the orthopaedic team play in the restoration and
rehabilitation of Mr Walters?

7 How might you help to relieve Mr Walters'
anxiety about his operation?

FURTHER READING

ARTHRITIS AND RHEUMATISM COUNCIL. *Rheumatoid Arthritis – A Handbook for Patients*. London: Arthritis and Rheumatism Council.

BARNES, C. G. 1978. 'Rheumatoid Arthritis – The Team Approach is the Answer.' *Nursing Mirror*, **147** (22): 30–5.

BROWN-SKEERS, V. 1979. 'How The Nurse Practitioner Manages the Rheumatoid Arthritis Patient.' *Nursing (Horsham)*, **9** (6): 26–35.

HART, F. D. 1981. 'Rheumatology: Osteoarthritis and Rheumatoid Arthritis.' *Nursing Mirror*, **153** (20) Supp: ii–v.

PANAYI, G. S. (Ed.) 1980. *Essential Rheumatology for Nurses and Therapists*. Eastbourne, Sussex: Baillière Tindall.

SWINSON, D. R. & SWINBURN, W. R. 1980. *Rheumatology*. Sevenoaks: Hodder and Stoughton.

7

David Spooner, who sustains a comminuted fracture of his lower leg in a motorcycle accident

HISTORY

David Spooner, aged 20 years, lives at home with his parents and his sister. He works as a tyre inspector at a well known tyre-making company. He enjoys his work and rides to work on a motorcycle from his home five miles away.

One evening, after eating his dinner, he left home telling his parents he was going to meet his mates.

Riding along a country road David lost control and fell off his bike. He found that he could not move his left leg and blood was seeping through his trousers.

Fortunately another motorcyclist came along the road soon after the accident and after checking that David was all right, he sped off to call for the police and an ambulance.

They both arrived promptly. The ambulance men put a dressing on David's left leg and immobilised it in a plastic splint. The policeman took road measurements and collected David's belongings. David was taken to the local Accident and Emergency Department.

ADMISSION TO THE HOSPITAL

On arrival he was welcomed by Linda. She helped David onto the trolley, and quickly took routine baseline observations. She called

What is an open comminuted fracture? A fracture is a break in the continuity of the bone.
Comminuted means broken in more than two pieces.
Open means that the bone has pierced the skin and is exposed to the air.
It is sometimes called a compound fracture.

the Casulty Officer to see him. During the examination the doctor asked David what happened at the scene of the accident. He ascertained that David had not lost consciousness and he found extensive bruising on his arms and grazing on his left hand. The doctor helped Linda to cut away his trousers to see the damage to his left leg. There was a thigh laceration and an open comminuted fracture of the left tibia and fibula with extensive skin loss.

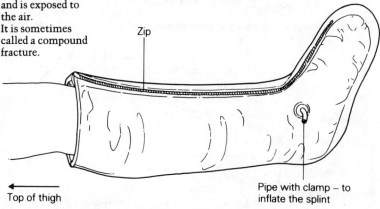

Zip

Top of thigh

Pipe with clamp – to inflate the splint

Immobilisation at scene of accident with a plastic splint

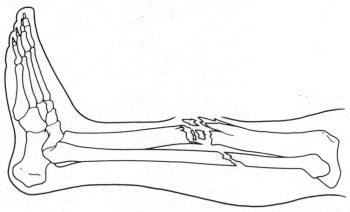

An open comminuted fracture

The doctor sent David for chest and abdominal X-rays to see if he had any internal injuries. He was accompanied by Linda who explained what was going to happen and held his hand. David was very frightened by the sight of the wound. He asked, 'Am I going to lose my leg, nurse?' Linda reassured him by explaining that many observations and tests would be taken and that everything would be done to save his leg. David was also very worried about his job. Linda said that she would telephone his employer as soon as possible and explain why he would not be at work.

An X-ray of his leg was also taken to assess the complete damage. Blood was taken for tests of haemoglobin, group and cross matching, as he had lost a lot of blood and would need a transfusion.

NURSING CARE

Initial stages

He was in great pain. He was given an intramuscular injection of Pethidine Hydrochloride for the pain and another of Benethamine Penicillin (Triplopen), which is a broad spectrum antibiotic, to prevent the spread of infection. David also had an injection of tetanus toxoid as he could not remember if he had been immunised before. This injection is to prevent David developing Tetanus by stimulating the production of antitoxins. Booster doses are required to produce active immunity. An injection of Humotet, an anti-tetanus immunoglobin, was also given to provide immediate protection until the tetanus toxoid takes effect.

The anaesthetist inquired when David last had something to eat or drink as he would have to have a general anaesthetic before reducing his fracture.

Linda verified that David had signed his consent form and was wearing an identity band. Then she went to determine whether someone had managed to notify his parents.

When Linda telephoned Mr and Mrs Spooner she informed them of what had happened to David and that he would require surgery. They were very anxious and said they would come straight away to the Accident and Emergency Department. Linda did not discourage them as it was not far for them to come and David would not be going to theatre until 10.30 p.m., four hours after he had last eaten.

That evening David was taken to the operating theatre where his wound was scrubbed out with a sterile nail brush to remove any micro-organisms that could cause complications. The skin was cleaned with hydrogen peroxide and covered with a sterile dressing.

After reduction of his fractures his leg was immobilised using an external fixator. The pins hold the fracture fragments and these in turn are held in place by the external pins.

An external fixator

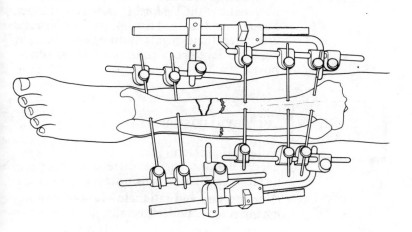

Rehabilitation

David returned from his operation to the recovery area where he stayed the rest of the night.

In the morning he was transferred to the orthopaedic trauma ward. He was welcomed by Christine, the ward nurse, and his bed was wheeled into a four bedded bay. David was very quiet. He looked pale.

Jill, the recovery nurse, explained to Christine what had taken place and how his wound had been treated. She also mentioned to Christine that David had not asked many questions about his leg or the external fixator. During the night his observations had fluctuated. As a falling blood pressure and rising pulse denote that he may be about to enter shock or may be haemorrhaging (which might lead to shock), frequent observations had been taken. Now, however, his readings had returned to more normal values. Observations were now to be taken four-hourly. He had also passed 350 ml of urine since the operation. There was an IV infusion sited in his right arm which would need careful observation.

Christine noticed that the end of the bed was elevated and the leg further raised on a pillow. She checked the pedal pulse in both legs and compared them regularly to ensure that any signs of developing complications would be noted.

for David postoperatively

Potential problem The fracture site releases fat droplets into the bloodstream and they may occlude capillaries, causing fat embolism.

Nursing care and rationale Be aware of any changes in David especially after 72 hours have passed. Inform the doctor immediately if he shows any of the following which may indicate the presence of fat embolism:

Confusion

Drowsiness

Breathlessness

Rapid pulse

Skin haemorrhage over chest and shoulders ('petechial rash')

Elevated temperature

Fat embolism can occur because fat droplets are released into the blood stream from the bone marrow at the fracture site. These droplets are then carried to the lungs where they cause occlusion of the capillaries. The patient becomes breathless due to the defective exchange of gases. Drowsiness and confusion are due to cerebral anoxia. This problem is most likely to occur in the first 72 hours following the accident.

Evaluation David did not develop any of the above signs, apart from a slightly elevated temperature on the second day.

Potential problem Venous stasis leading to deep vein thrombosis may occur as a complication of enforced bed rest and must be prevented.

Nursing care and rationale David will be seen by Mary, the physiotherapist, twice daily for an active exercise programme. Report any pain and tenderness in his calf and any inability to move his foot. Due to inactivity of muscle, venous congestion can arise. This in turn can lead to a clot (thrombus) forming. This thrombus can then become detached and occlude a vein, possibly leading to an embolus causing death, e.g. pulmonary embolism.

Evaluation David enjoyed doing his exercises. They occupied his time and he felt he was keeping fit.

Actual problem The external fixator used to

maintain alignment of the fracture is heavy and awkward to move as the protruding pins catch frequently on bedclothes, etc. It allows the skin wound to heal either by being dressed or exposed to the air.

Nursing care and rationale Explain to David that the external fixator allows the skin wounds of the injured leg to heal by being uncovered and that the pins are holding the fracture in place. The pins sites must be watched for redness and oozing. Unless otherwise ordered by the doctor, the sites remain intact and untouched to prevent the risk of infection tracking to the bone (osteomyelitis).

David can move his leg normally but carefully as hitting the pins will hurt. Also warn David that the external fixator is heavy and that he will find it difficult to move his leg until he gets used to it.

During the day, David can place his leg on a pillow. At night a bed cradle will help to keep the bedclothes off his leg.

Encourage David to read books and listen to the radio to counteract boredom from inactivity. Wheel him out into the day room in his bed to watch the television. Use a wheelchair with elevated leg pieces to go to the bathroom. Persuade David's relatives to take him around the hospital in his wheelchair; this helps to maintain his dignity and independence. Assist David to accept his temporary altered body image by encouraging him to pursue his hobbies and interests within his limitations as without this his rehabilitation will be slow.

Examine the colour, sensation, warmth and movements of the ankle and observe for any swelling.

Compare the pedal pulses as the pins go through the tissues and could cause compression of blood vessels and/or nerves. Any impairment will cause pain and ischaemia.

Evaluation David found the external fixator

frightening at first. He was worried about moving his leg and amazed at how heavy it was and how awkward to move around. He found it much easier when the swelling of the whole leg had gone down. Turning in bed required great care to avoid catching the pins on the bed clothes. The bed cradle took care of this difficulty at night, and during the day he lay on top of his bed with no bedding over his leg.

David enjoyed being pushed around in his bed. About two weeks after his injury he went out to wash at the sink using the wheelchair. However, he was very worried that someone might bump into him. He played cards and Scrabble with other patients on the ward. His family and friends visited frequently but he did not like them to look at his leg, as he thought that they might be upset at seeing all the pins going through it.

Actual problem   He is anxious about his job and money and these worries will hinder his rehabilitation.

Nursing care and rationale   Inform David of all procedures. Contact his personnel officer at work and ask him to visit. Information and reassurance by the firm itself will allow David to be less anxious. Every effort can then be channelled towards his rehabilitation.

Evaluation   David had been informed that it would take about 6 to 12 weeks for his leg to heal. The personnel officer came to see him and explained he would get his full pay for up to six months.

Actual problem   The immobility will make it difficult for David to maintain his personal hygiene.

Nursing care and rationale   Help David to wash his left foot. He can use a wheelchair with extended leg pieces to go to wash at the sink. Mobility prevents pressure sores developing and maintains an intact skin, as well as fostering his feelings of independence.

Evaluation   David found it difficult to wash his left foot as he was unable to reach it due to the bulkiness of the external fixator. He was worried that water would get into his wound and lead to infection.

Potential problem   Constipation may arise as a result of enforced bed rest and it is important to promote normal bowel habits.

Nursing care and rationale   Using David's menu card, help him choose foods high in fibre, e.g. bran, fruit, and vegetables. Encourage him to drink at least 3 litres of fluid a day.

Evaluation   David found he disliked bran intensely but enjoyed the prunes and custard which his mother brought in for him. He drank plenty of lemonade and coca-cola.

After 6 weeks the doctor reviewed David's situation. An X-ray of his left leg showed that the fracture was healing. Pleased with this progress the doctor told him that the external fixator would be removed under general anaesthetic and the leg immobilised in a functional brace. Though his fracture is stable, it is not yet strong enough to bear his full body weight.

David was prepared for the operating theatre in the normal way. In theatre he had his external fixator removed under general anaesthetic. Plaster of Paris was moulded to his thigh as far down as the knee. Hinges were then inserted and the moulding continued from below the knee to his ankle.

Other materials can be used to make the brace; some are made of thermoplastic with metal hinges. This type is removable for washing the leg. As it sets very quickly the patient can walk straight after its application.

When David returned to the ward he was awake and delighted with his new cast. The plaster of Paris had to dry first before David could start mobilisation (see pp. 40, 41).

What is a functional brace?
This is a method of immobilising a limb by compressing the tissues evenly throughout the length of the fracture, but allowing movement at joints above and below it. Therefore the brace must fit snugly to be effective.

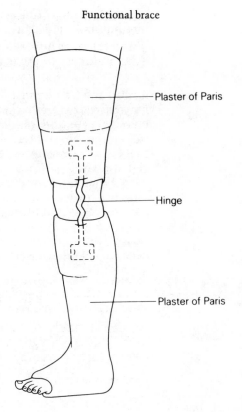

Functional brace

Plaster of Paris

Hinge

Plaster of Paris

CARE PLAN

for David in his functional brace

Actual problem David must be immobile until his functional brace dries (about 48 hours).

Nursing care and rationale Explain to him that heat will be felt as the plaster of Paris dries (for up to 72 hours). Inspect the cast for any rough edges. Examine the foot and knee for warmth, colour, swelling, sensation and movement. Too tight a brace causes constrictions of the blood vessels while too loose a brace is ineffectual.

Evaluation The functional brace was well moulded to David's thigh and lower leg. He did not complain of any pain or rough edges.

Actual problem The left leg will have lost some muscle tone after its period of immobilisation and David must follow a new exercise programme to improve it.

Nursing care and rationale Exercises with Mary, the physiotherapist, should be done twice daily. Encourage quadriceps exercises and straight leg exercises as demonstrated on p. 70. When he can walk, David is to use elbow crutches for balance, though he is allowed to put his full weight through his leg.

Ensure that the functional brace is well fitting. Restoration of functional activity is necessary so that David can continue regaining his independence.

Evaluation David worked hard at his exercise programme as he wanted to get up and walk again. He found that at first his knee was swollen at the end of the day. Until he got used to the different weight of the functional brace, he kept hitting his other leg with the hinge.

NURSING CARE

Planning discharge

David worked hard at his knee exercises and soon got used to his crutches. He enjoyed going to the Occupational Therapy Department to use the bicycle fretsaw and the treadle lathe. These are used to increase the range of movement and strengthen the lower limbs. He was allowed home when he could bend his knee to 90 degrees and was able to manage stairs.

His parents were delighted that he had done so well. Eight weeks after his accident he was discharged home.

It was 10 weeks after seeing his personnel officer that he went back to work, mainly in the office until he felt strong enough to do a bit more.

At 12 weeks he had an outpatients' appointment, and his functional brace was removed. His skin was dry and flaky. Arachis oil was applied to the skin and soon made it soft and smooth. Another exercise programme was planned by the physiotherapist until he could bend his knee and ankle. Four months later he was back at his work as a tyre inspector and riding his motorbike.

TEST YOURSELF

1 What care did David require before going to the operating theatre?

2 What were David's needs after his fracture had been immobilised and how did the nurse care for him?

3 What did the nurse have to be aware of when a fracture is immobilised in an external fixator and why?

4 Which members of the team played a role in David's care?

5 What problems, if any, did David encounter with his functional brace?

6 What plans were made to cope with David's boredom?

FURTHER READING

APLEY, A. J. AND SOLOMON, L. 1982. *Apley's System of Orthopaedics and Fractures*, 6th ed. London: Butterworth Scientific.
BETTS-SYMONDS, G. 1982. Functional Bracing of Fractures of the Tibia and Fibula. *Nursing Times* 78 (50): 2123–6.
GROUT, *et al.* 1979. Hoffman Apparatus – Boning up on a Brace. *Nursing Mirror* 149 (16): 46–9.
STEEL-NICHOLSON, A. 1984. The Belfast Fixator. *Nursing Times* 80 (8): 53–6.

8 Aftercare

Going home from hospital is a wonderful feeling. Full of anticipation of what can and is to be done sets high hopes for the future. The patient reassures himself with the thought, 'I must be better or I would not be allowed home.'

Yet there are several traps awaiting the patient at home:

Coping with the daily routine of every day tasks
Pain (which probably still remains)
Moving about the house
Returning to work

No matter how much the patient and the members of the orthopaedic team have planned the discharge, life at home is different from life in hospital. In hospital it was, 'Up and dressed by 9 a.m. and off to the Physiotherapy Department. Cup of coffee at 10.30 a.m. and back to the exercise class. Return to the ward for lunch and a rest before setting off to the Occupational Therapy Department in the afternoon.' This left the evening free for watching television and chatting to relatives and patients.

Yet at home housework, shopping and meals to be prepared become part of the day to day existence and loom large in the patient's mind, becoming of paramount importance. The patient often becomes alarmed that so much energy is required to perform each small task. He becomes tired, irritable, exhausted and possibly constantly aware of a niggling pain. He then becomes depressed, fearing that he is losing his independence which he fought so hard to regain during those long weeks in hospital.

Each patient's perception of pain varies to a greater or lesser extent depending on the type of pain. A sudden intense pain resulting from some traumatic injury (breaking a bone in an accident) is often relieved by the administration of a narcotic drug. The patient copes well with this acute pain as she knows that it will subside as soon as the drug takes effect. As the healing process progresses, the acute pain sensation declines and she feels that she is improving. However the healing process can bring its own complications, e.g. deep scar formation within the tissues, leading to the dull ache of chronic pain that is with the patient constantly as the weeks and months go by. Patients are usually released from hospital before the healing process is complete and this chronic pain will continue at home. As has been recognised in previous chapters, medication taken regularly will help to relieve this pain. However the patient may not recognise the importance of taking regular analgesia. A change in position may help relieve the pain (such as lying down as opposed to sitting). Yet the patient may not want to move for fear of setting off the pain again.

Wandering about the house and manoeuvring in between the furniture becomes a major operation if the patient has an appliance. Appliances are bulky and not very malleable. It might be easier to either remove some furniture from the room or place it against the walls, until the appliance can be manipulated with skill.

Certain points are worth considering:

1 Moving into one room for a while
2 Planning frequent rest periods between tasks

3   Remember that exercises taught by the physiotherapist and the activities shown by the occupational therapist complement one another, e.g. peeling vegetables is good for wrist action (exercise) as well as fulfilling the need for food (activity of daily living).
4   Muscle bulk and tone increases with exercise. Stamina for coping with daily activities is built up and zest for life returns.

This is probably a good time for seeing the General Practitioner with a view to returning to work. If it is at all possible, working for 2 or 3 days a week helps alleviate the stress of returning to full time exployment after weeks or months off work.

INDEX